'A magnificent book that is rich in clinical material and a must-read for (mental) health care professionals, many of whom will recognise their own childhood history of parentification and the far-reaching consequences of it.'

Prof. Em. Dr Nel Draijer, *emeritus associate professor of Psychiatry, University of Amsterdam (NL), psychologist, psychotherapist and psychoanalyst.*

'It was Boszormeny-Nagy who originally defined the concept of parentification, but it is definitely Kinet who masterfully deconstructs, enriches and revitalises it in his new book. Marvellously written and full of clinical wisdom, this book is a must-read for every clinician working in the fields of psychotherapy, psychiatry and psychoanalysis.'

Prof. Dr Benedicte Lowyck, *clinical psychologist and associate professor at KU Leuven (BE).*

Mark Kinet offers a profound exploration of parentification, weaving together psychoanalytic and systemic thinking with remarkable clarity. His gripping narratives and intellectual depth make this work a touchstone for anyone seeking to grasp the full complexity of this phenomenon.

Prof. Dr Peter Rober, *Professor at KU Leuven (BE) and author of* Becoming an Effective Family Therapist (Routledge, 2024)

Parentification is an invisible yet profoundly influential force that shapes the emotional lives of many people. Mark Kinet takes the reader on a comprehensive journey into this concept, moving between psychoanalytic theory, systemic thinking, attachment research, and clinical practice. A rich and empathetic work that is indispensable for clinicians, researchers, and anyone who wants to understand – and change – the hidden dimensions of family life.

Prof. Dr Nicole Vliegen, *Professor at KU Leuven (BE), psychoanalytic child psychotherapist and psychoanalyst*

'He did it again. Mark Kinet knows better than anyone how to connect an essential phenomenon from clinical practice with the history of the theory formation surrounding it. This book focuses on the suffering caused by parentification. The traces of this traumatic process can be found in "ghosts in the nursery", present in internalised object representations, fantasies or through neuropsychoanalytic mechanisms. With his many case studies, Kinet once again touches on the core of psychoanalytic work: "understanding and working through the parent's inner history.'

Prof. Em. Dr Frans Schalkwijk, *emeritus professor at the University of Amsterdam (NL), psychoanalyst, and former editor-in-chief of Tijdschrift voor Psychoanalyse (Dutch Journal of Psychoanalysis).*

'Drawing on both systemic and psychoanalytic perspectives, Mark Kinet offers a compelling and comprehensive account of parentification. With vivid and lucid prose, he weaves together rich theoretical reflections and finely nuanced clinical insights. For anyone seeking to understand parentification from multiple angles—its manifestations in children and adult patients, and its relevance to choosing a psychotherapeutic vocation—this book is an essential read.'

Prof. Dr Reitske Meganck, *associate professor of clinical psychology and psychoanalysis at Ghent University (BE) and a psychoanalytic psychotherapist in private practice.*

'When children grow up too soon, something essential is lost—and something enduring is formed. In this profound psychoanalytic study, Mark Kinet traces how parentification quietly shapes personality, attachment, vocation, and suffering across a lifetime. Drawing on rich clinical material and the full depth of psychoanalytic theory, this book reveals parentification as both a hidden wound and a powerful, fate-shaping force in adult psychic life.'

Prof. Dr Damiaan Denys, psychiatrist and philosopher, Professor of Psychiatry at the University of Amsterdam (NL)

The Psychodynamics and Psychogenesis of Parentification

Why do some of us grow up too soon and spend a lifetime caring for others at the cost of ourselves? In this deeply humane study, psychiatrist and psychoanalyst **Mark Kinet** explores *parentification*: the invisible role reversal in which children become their parents' caretakers, confidants, or even partners.

Blending vivid clinical portraits, psychoanalytic depth, and literary sensibility, Kinet traces how early caregiving shapes our psychic architecture and builds resilience, but also leaves enduring fractures. Drawing on Freud, Ferenczi, Balint, Klein, Winnicott, Bion, Kernberg, Kohut, Bowlby, Fonagy, and Lacan, as well as infant research and contemporary neuropsychoanalysis, he reconstructs the unconscious history of the 'wise baby,' the 'wounded healer,' and the adult child who cannot stop repairing others. Across richly textured chapters and cinematic intermezzos, Kinet interweaves theory and therapy, empathy and analysis. He demonstrates how psychoanalytic work can transform the 'inherited' burden of parentification into creative care.

Written with clarity and compassion, *The Psychodynamics and Psychogenesis of Parentification* is both a clinical study and a meditation on the human need to give and be given to. It speaks to therapists, scholars, and all readers seeking to understand the paradox of 'loving' too much and too early.

Mark Kinet is a psychiatrist, psychotherapist, and psychoanalyst based in Belgium. He is the author of *The Spirit of the Drive in Neuropsychoanalysis* (2023), *Psychoanalytic Principles in Psychiatric Practice: A Remedy by Truth* (2024), *Psychoanalytic Psychotherapy in Psychiatric Practice: Premises and Clinical Portraits* (2025) and *Patient Testimonies of Psychodynamic Psychotherapy: Reported and Recorded* (2025).

The Psychodynamics and Psychogenesis of Parentification

Mark Kinet

Routledge
Taylor & Francis Group
LONDON AND NEW YORK

Designed cover image: © Courtesy Steven Peters Caraballo, The Red, oil on linen, 50 x 40 cm, 2022

First published 2027
by Routledge
4 Park Square, Milton Park, Abingdon, Oxon OX14 4RN

and by Routledge
605 Third Avenue, New York, NY 10158

Routledge is an imprint of the Taylor & Francis Group, an informa business

British Library Cataloguing-in-Publication Data
A catalogue record for this book is available from the British Library

Library of Congress Cataloging-in-Publication Data
A catalog record has been requested for this book

ISBN: 978-1-041-08510-2 (hbk)
ISBN: 978-1-041-08509-6 (pbk)
ISBN: 978-1-003-64572-6 (ebk)

DOI: 10.4324/9781003645726

Typeset in Times New Roman
by Taylor & Francis Books

Contents

Chapter 1

Prelude

The Red

(poem for the cover painting by Steven Peters Caraballo)

This costume sings opera rather than stage.
Warm to the eye, a velvet flame,
Touched with baroque, a festive guise,
Dressed for a night, it speaks, disguised.
Red, colour of passion and fire,
Of love's first bloom, of raw desire,
Of battle, of fury and fight,
A flash of danger, of stops in the night.

The pose, perhaps too still,
Like a vase, longing to be filled,
A vessel of shadow and gleam.
A box of secrets, a smuggler's dream,
A flask for a breath that hides and hums,
A pulse where something silent drums.

A shape reminding one of princely grace,
The linen collar frames a face
That listens, childlike, calm, and wise —
A quiet ear for words that bite.

Mark Kinet

DOI: 10.4324/9781003645726-1

Chapter 2

Overture

Charles

The Red Boy is a famous portrait painted exactly 200 years ago by Sir Thomas Lawrence. It portrays Charles Lambton, the elder son of John Lambton (later created Earl of Durham), at age seven. The cover image of this book is titled *The Red*. The artist Steven Peters Caraballo made Charles vanish. All that remains is the somewhat posh costume of what appears to be a boy. The viewer has to fill in the contours. The pose is poised and, in a way, dramatic, so I guess Charles is a good pseudonym to start with for a clinical case.[1]

Charles, in his thirties, presents himself for clinical psychotherapy. Since the age of eighteen, he has been in treatment with two successive psychiatrists and has undergone both individual and couples therapy with three different psychologists. He begins by saying, 'I feel anxious in relationships, especially with friends. I constantly need reassurance and fear rejection. I work very hard.' He then begins to talk spontaneously about his father. 'I have a lot of anger towards him. I had a turbulent youth.' He also speaks of an older brother who was diagnosed with autism spectrum disorder and who placed a great deal of pressure on the family. The father couldn't cope. Charles's parents divorced during his adolescence. His father ended up in psychiatric care and was eventually diagnosed with borderline personality disorder. He had also struggled with alcohol dependence for years, though with the help of AA, he has now been sober for quite some time.

The father was reportedly largely absent from the child-rearing. He was emotionally disengaged. Though he worked in the therapeutic field himself and enjoyed a certain status and respect there, he has been on long-term disability for years. Charles describes him as narcissistic. 'He likes to present himself as important, but he offers little space to others.' According to Charles, his father thinks in black-and-white terms, dividing people into the good and the bad. He lacks perspective. His mother is a few years older than his father. Charles describes her as loving and caring, yet also very emotional and clingy. At times, he finds her manipulative. He feels he

DOI: 10.4324/9781003645726-2

always has to read between the lines. He describes his relationship with her as 'symbiotic.'

Charles (who is himself a care professional) refers to himself as 'a textbook example of parentification':

> I was drawn into raising my two brothers and my little sister. My mother did her best, but she had her own difficulties. She has been on antidepressants for years. She is insecure and has always tried to erase herself. The same was expected of me. I had to work hard to be seen or to be loved. It's exhausting. It has made me depressed. I'm tired—or tired of it. Lately, my anger has been surfacing more often.

When asked about his development, Charles says he was very anxious and insecure during primary school. In his own words, he never really found his footing. He went through a turbulent adolescence. He skated avidly and felt 'special, different.' He stole at school, skipped classes, and enjoyed partying—by which he means drinking and smoking cannabis. He had a lot of mixed feelings—he felt rebellious, yet also 'very compassionate' towards his mother. He was especially angry with his father and sent him many accusatory emails during that period.

He had his first girlfriend, slightly older than him, from ages fourteen to seventeen. She ended the relationship 'for older boys.' He later had a ten-year relationship with Suzanne. They lived together and bought a house. 'It was an unhealthy relationship. I took care of her. She was dominant and manipulative. She used to throw notes with instructions on the floor for me to pick up. She made me feel like a loser.' After he left her, she continued to pursue him for a long time. Emotionally and financially, he paid a steep price—she made him suffer and pay excessively. At the time of his admission, he had been in a relationship with his current partner for several years, who, like him, works in the healthcare field. They now have two children together.

Charles completed university studies and works in youth care as a residential group supervisor. He also conducts therapy in private practice—partly out of financial necessity, as he had debts with both his ex and his current wife. He underwent about six months of clinical psychotherapy, first as an inpatient and later in day treatment. Since then, he has been attending weekly psychotherapy sessions for around three years. I will refer back to him and his psychoanalytic process at the end of this book.[2]

From the fact that Charles describes himself as a textbook example of parentification, one might assume he knows what's wrong. But nothing could be further from the truth. Analogically, many of us may intellectually understand that our parents (and, by extension, our intimate circle) leave a mark on who we have become. But only a thorough psychoanalysis reveals to what extent—and with what consequences—it is the case.

In Charles's story, parentification is glaringly obvious. Some elements are plainly visible: his caregiving role towards his siblings, the paternal void, and the emotionally needy mother to whom he was very close. Later in the book, I will elaborate on the general advantages and disadvantages of parentification, as well as its constructive and destructive forms. It can be instrumental or emotional, and in the latter case, may manifest either consciously or unconsciously. For the child (within the adult), it leads—like any symptom—to both gains and losses, pleasure and pain, and more specifically to an illusion of importance that paradoxically is not in the child's own best interest. There is both a lack[3] (often a cocktail of abandonment anxiety, depression, and rage) and an excessive burden of care that, sooner or later, takes its toll. From a kind of destructive entitlement, love, care, and attention are later demanded or extracted from 'innocent' others, from whom unreasonable restitution is expected. Parentification can also lead to a kind of exhaustion or burnout due to chronic stress and strain on the brain.

All of this can be understood as the result of a vertical (rather than horizontal) splitting of the psyche. It may be compared to the two sides of the moon: one (sunny side up) exposed to daylight, while the dark side remains perpetually hidden. This corresponds, respectively, to the parental and child aspects of the self—the therapist's side and the patient's side. While the child may have seemed precocious and mature, childish or infantile traits increasingly emerge—often inappropriately—causing misunderstanding, if not rejection or condemnation, from the intimate environment. Behind the façade of normality—or even high functioning—unseen needs come to light, both literally and figuratively. This may occur gradually or suddenly, like a bolt from the blue. This brief and superficial sketch of phenomenology and manifestations conceals, upon closer inspection, a complex interplay of psychodynamic and psychogenetic factors that often remain underexplored in the literature on parentification and which this book aims to examine in depth.

I begin with a discussion of the history and concept of parentification and its various degrees and forms. It is an important pathogenic factor in all kinds of psychopathology. In clinical reality it is almost always more or less complexly mixed with other etiological components. It rarely manifests itself in its 'pure' form. First, a very common form of parentification is discussed separately: that typically seen in adult children of alcoholic parents. The following chapter will discuss the obvious necessity of an integrated, systemic, and psychoanalytic approach to these kinds of problems. The next chapter, 'Curiously Called,' is specifically dedicated to parentification, as it is often found in the therapeutic calling/vocation of the so-called wounded healer. In the next and—by far—longest chapter, the emphasis will be on the unconscious psychogenesis and psychodynamic structure of parentification. The following are addressed in succession: Freud's rescue fantasies; Ferenczi's wise baby and identification with the aggressor; Balint's basic fault; Klein's envious, manic, and obsessional reparations; Winnicott's False Self; Kernberg's identity diffusion and sadistic superego; Kohut's self-object functions taken up by the child; Bion's reversed alpha function and the container-contained dynamic; Bowlby's pre-occupied or disorganised attachment; Fonagy's alien self and counter-productive hyper-mentalisation; infant research perspectives on parentification; the neuropsychoanalysis of parentification; and finally Lacan's failed triangulation and paternal function. To illustrate all this clinically, several intermezzos present cases both of overt and hidden parentification, within neurotic or narcissistic/borderline structures, among both outpatients and inpatients.

Under the heading 'Fatefully Yours!' all these threads are brought together in a final reflection. As in my previous books and as in the Prelude, I remain committed to opera—more specifically, *open* opera, or *opera aperta*.[4] Every interpretation is at its best when it remains transitional and unsaturated.[5] It offers a container into which the patient can insert or rediscover their own meanings. Hence, my choice of the title Overture rather than the more conventional Prologue.

Notes

1 Potentially personally identifying information presented that relates directly or indirectly to an individual, or individuals, has been changed throughout this book to disguise and safeguard the confidentiality, privacy, and data protection rights of those concerned, in accordance with the usual psychoanalytic journal's anonymisation policies.
2 See my trilogy on psychodynamic psychiatry with Routledge for an elaborated and extensive presentation of my working models and methods.
3 Throughout the book, the word 'lack' will be used for a varying amalgam of deficiency, lack, or shortage. Let me put the blame on Jacques Lacan, aka Jack the Lack. To him, this lack is structurally inherent to human/symbolic language, but it is quantitatively and qualitatively different for each of us (Fink, 1995, pp 54–59).
4 Freud's work definitely belongs to the category of *opera aperta* (Eco, 1962).
5 Winnicott (1951) and Ferro (2002, p. 23), respectively, the last one referring to Bion: 'The analyst's task is to make interpretations that are sufficiently unsaturated to allow the field to evolve; they must stimulate rather than define meaning.'

References

Eco, U. (1962). *The Open Work*, translated by Anna Cancogni with an Introduction by David Robey. Cambridge, MA: Harvard UP, 1989.

Ferro, A. (2002). Narrative derivatives of the analytic field. *International Journal of Psycho-Analysis*, 83 (4), 807–818.

Fink, B. (1995). *The Lacanian Subject: Between Language and Jouissance*. Princeton, NJ: Princeton University Press.

Winnicott, D. W. (1951). Transitional objects and transitional phenomena. *Through Paediatrics to Psycho-analysis* (pp. 229–242). London: Hogarth, 1958.

Chapter 3

Parentification Introduced

History and Concept

The Unconscious as History

I will start with two well-known statements about history. One: history teaches us that we do not learn from our history.[1] Two: those who do not know their history are doomed to repeat it.[2] If there is one premise that characterises my psychoanalytical work, it is the historical one. A classic distinction is made between prehistory and history. Prehistory refers to the period before writing. All knowledge about prehistory must be based on archaeological finds: the famous 'stones and bones,' i.e. tools, bones, cave paintings, traces of habitation. History only begins when written sources are available. Fragments of clay tablets, papyri, inscriptions or chronicles create a body of written tradition. They allow events, forms of society, and ideas to be reconstructed more directly.[3]

Despite all its conceptual eccentricities, psychoanalysis is actually very simple. Our feelings and (over)sensitivities do not come out of thin air, nor are they written in the stars. Rather, they have to do with the constellation of characters from which or under which we were born, as well as with what we have experienced positively or negatively along the way and have 'made' or 'learned' to be 'right' or 'wrong.' Freud's Id may be called a drive system, but his unconscious is primarily a memory system.[4] It consists roughly of implicit or procedural memory and explicit or biographical memory.[5] The former is expressed in the repetition of our actions. Our (inter)actions are its silent witnesses. Only the latter can we recount and retell in various ways. The history we write in this way is not static but dynamic. At first, we write it in a rather two-dimensional way. Initially, our universe is animistic and still populated by mythological/fairytale figures. Only later does it become more nuanced and three-dimensional. It acquires a more truthful character. However, it varies depending on the perspective from which we start and depending on the audience (including ourselves) to whom we address it. Its editors use the linguistic interventions that characterise both dream work and (conversely) analytical work, respectively, to conceal and to reveal.[6]

DOI: 10.4324/9781003645726-3

This (subjective) *historiography* is therefore essentially (not fact or fiction but) *faction.*

Following my previous books published by Routledge (the first on neuropsychoanalysis and then my trilogy on psychodynamic psychiatry), I will now discuss parentification.[7] It is a term or concept that is particularly often used in relation to children and young people and by family or systemic therapists. It refers to a largely macroscopically observable phenomenon in which the child becomes a 'parent' too quickly and in which the roles are reversed for various forms of care. In my long career as an adult psychiatrist, I have gradually come to recognise the phenomenon of parentification as an extremely prevalent aetiopathogenic factor. It plays an invisible and misunderstood (leading) role in many psychological problems in adults. As will become apparent, I will start at the surface and peel away the layers of parentification until we finally reach its deepest core and can contemplate it in its complex, multidimensional form. Psychoanalysis does not attempt to reduce psychological complexity, but rather to (help) express it.

The Concept

Parentification is a term mainly used by family therapists and social workers who work with children and/or young people. It primarily concerns more or less visible (interaction) patterns in which the child becomes 'trapped.' It is a process of expectations and role distribution within a family system, in which the target is chosen according to complex determinants, usually by the entire system. This choice is determined by previous phases of family relationships and the development of each family member. Family members sometimes take turns in the parentified role. However, the more unshakeable this division of roles is, the more problems it will cause in the parentified child's development. Based on their highly developed sensitivity and caring abilities, the child fulfils a 'superior' role within the family. These qualities, combined with the parents' dependence, also give the child a strong position of power within the system. In a first definition, it is therefore a process in which the child takes on the emotional or logistical needs of the parent(s) or the family, thereby neglecting or being neglected in their own needs.

Parentification is more common in families with psychosocial vulnerabilities, such as divorce,[8] mental or physical illness of a parent,[9] addiction problems,[10] or a migrant background.[11] Situational and cultural factors also play a role: in collectivist societies such as parts of Asia, parentification is more often perceived as normal or valuable.[12] In Western contexts, on the other hand, parentification is more likely to be seen as a violation of psychological boundaries between parent and child, with potential risks for the development of the self and separation-individuation. Difficult socio-economic circumstances increase the risk of parentification.[13] Usually, the oldest child is chosen for parentification.[14] Girls are more easily parentified than boys.[15] The child may be 'promoted' to a surrogate partner. This is referred to as spousification. This phenomenon is more common in single-parent families. Mother-son spousification is more common than father-daughter spousification.[16] For example, the mother may prefer her son over other men because she feels safer with him (including sexually).

A distinction is often made between instrumental and emotional parentification.[17] In the former, the child takes care of and is responsible for specific tasks that contribute to the family's physical survival, such as caring for younger siblings, shopping, cleaning, caring for a sick family member, or contributing to the family budget. Emotional parentification is more about the emotional or social needs of the parent(s) or family that need to be met. For example, the child may act as a confidant, a surrogate partner, or a mediator in marital or intra-family conflicts. Although these forms often occur together, they will have different effects. Emotional parentification is more often associated with negative psychological outcomes,[18] while instrumental parentification—provided it is age-appropriate—more often leads to positive competence development.[19]

This typology shows that the 'diagnosis' of parentification is initially based on previously visible manifestations. All the literature shows that emotional parentification has a more negative impact than instrumental parentification. This emotional variant is even compared to emotional neglect and is given the status of a cumulative traumatic experience with all the consequences that entail during adulthood,[20] not least in the form of fear of more intimate relationships later in life.[21]

Salvador Minuchin

In *Families of the Slums* (1976), Salvador Minuchin and his colleagues first mentioned the term 'parental child'. I quote: 'The vacuum in the family system created by the lack of parental functioning is filled by the attempted assumption of executive functions on the part of the parental child or children.'[22] In families of lower socio-economic status, it is common for the eldest child to take on parental responsibilities. In their view, this is an adaptive phenomenon that is characteristic of large families, single-parent families and families where one or both parents are often absent because of their job(s). These families can function well, and the parental child gains skills and independence.[23] There would therefore be no problem as long as the tasks are fairly distributed, age-appropriate, and recognised and appreciated.[24]

Minuchin, with his structuring of family therapy, is one of the all-time greats.[25] For him, families lie between two extremes: the tangled family and the loose sand family. In the tangled family, the boundaries between the subsystems are unclear, everyone knows everything about each other, and the behaviour of one family member directly influences that of others. There is a strong sense of togetherness at the expense of individual autonomy. This hinders the development of independence. In the loose-sand family, there are rigid boundaries between subsystems. If someone has problems here, it is hardly noticed by the other family members. As a result, a child will receive little support in developing independence. Between these two extremes lies what he calls homeostasis. This is a constantly shifting point at which the family maintains a healthy balance, allowing each individual to develop and flourish optimally. Minuchin worked as a psychiatrist in the fledgling state of Israel with refugee children and with juvenile delinquents from inner-city New York, among others. He trained in psychoanalysis in the Big Apple (1954–1967) but found the traditional psychoanalytic approach unsuitable for the patient population he was confronted with.[26]

Ivan Boszormenyi-Nagy

Parentification was only introduced as a separate concept after Minuchin, namely by the Hungarian-American psychiatrist Ivan Boszormenyi-Nagy.[27] With his transgenerational approach, he is considered the founder of the contextual approach in psychotherapy. He was inspired by both family therapy and psychoanalysis, particularly by one of its object-relations pioneers, Ronald Fairbairn.[28] Alice Van der Pas and Evert De Ruiter introduced the concept into the Dutch-speaking world.[29] According to all these authors, parentification refers to family circumstances in which the child is made responsible for the well-being of the parents. This contextual perspective could mistakenly give the impression that the child is merely passively subjected to such dynamics. However, from the outset, family therapists have been much more nuanced in their approach. 'It is a natural reflex for the therapist to respond to the child who is the scapegoat as if he or she were a victim who needs to be rescued from his or her oppressors. But it is more accurate to regard this 'victim' as a collaborator or even a winner.[30] The child may feel seduced and honoured by the implicit VIP status associated with parentification. In a sense, it therefore 'chooses' for itself: either for the creation or for the continuation of its impossible task. Of course, this 'choice' should be placed in quotation marks. After all, this is certainly not a voluntary and/or conscious choice. The 'privilege' they 'enjoy' is a trap because it involves a structural (rather than circumstantial) compulsion. This loyalty establishes an existential legacy. It is a commitment that protects the family at the expense of the individual's own development. A form of survivor's guilt can even occur when the child tries to break free. Every step towards self-expression can be unconsciously experienced as a form of crime, leading to the institutionalisation of an internal conflict between attachment and autonomy.

Boszormenyi-Nagy considers the behaviour of the 'parentifying' parent to be a form of symbiotic dependence. He distinguishes between two forms of this. There is functional dependence when the child takes on certain (often practical, organisational) tasks. This need not be detrimental and can even be seen as an exercise in responsibility. The condition is that the task assigned to the child is age-appropriate and that the child receives both mandate and recognition for fulfilling it. The direct consequences can even be described as positive. The child is seen as meaningful, as someone who makes a valuable contribution to the whole. This contributes to their self-definition (I am someone, I am seen, I exist) and sense of self-worth (I matter, I am valuable to myself and others). He contrasts this constructive form of parentification with the destructive form. The latter is more about dependence, in which the child is deprived of the opportunity to develop into an independent person. After all, they only 'serve' to fulfil their parents' deep needs. This latter form of dependence jeopardises the child's development and later adult functioning. The child becomes trapped in an existential loyalty to the parent figure. The child takes care of and is responsible for the parent. In doing so, it feels and acts grown up. However, as a carer, it becomes its own grandparent. At the same time, the child becomes a child of the account. Crucial to the pathological impact of parentification is that the parents deny or misrecognise this phenomenon. Destructive parentification blocks development. This can manifest itself in several areas: cognitively (e.g. studies are compromised), socially (more commitment to the family than enjoyment with peers), emotionally (depressed mood), and biologically (even growth retardation, delayed puberty). Self-sacrifice then becomes a real identity disorder. The child is trapped in the family system and can no longer escape from it 'with propriety'.

Italian family therapist Maurizio Andolfi strongly agrees with Boszormenyi-Nagy's views on parentification. He is certainly considered one of the most important authors in this field internationally.[31] Like Boszormenyi-Nagy, he emphasises that parentification does not (necessarily) have to be problematic. Children can play an active and competent role within the family. This promotes development, as the child learns empathy, responsibility, and a range of social skills. Only when the child has to permanently or exclusively take on the role of parent (parentification) or partner (spousification) without this being recognised as such does it burden or disrupt their own development. One tool he introduced to detect parentification and bring it to therapeutic attention is the genogram.[32] He considers it a map of the family world. It serves as a pertinent starting point in family therapy sessions to uncover intergenerational connections and emotional dynamics. It serves as a graphic map of family patterns. Andolfi uses it together with the children as an active guide, promoting open reflection and challenging stereotypical family narratives.

Alice Van der Pas

In Dutch-language literature, Alice Van der Pas, like Boszormenyi-Nagy and Minuchin, mentions crossing the generational line as a characteristic of parentification.[33] She considers parentification exclusively as a pathological process. She believes that parentification stems from a rejection of the child in childhood. According to her, the process is largely unconscious and is driven by deep-rooted emotional desires in both parent and child. The child is rejected when it appeals to the parent for affection, guidance, or support. On the other hand, it is accepted when it offers all of this to the parent. The parent lets the child know through their reactions that parental behaviour is preferred over age-appropriate behaviour. Van der Pas explicitly states that this concerns behaviour beyond the child's comprehension and that the child cannot properly control. The child inevitably fails in its parental role. At the same time, it is not accepted as a child. Yet the child protests little or not at all. It even resists change. On the one hand, we can compare this to the Stockholm syndrome described by Nils Bejerot, in which hostages sympathise with their captors.[34] Here, the defence mechanism of identification with the aggressor comes into play.[35] But the child may also feel flattered by the position of responsibility. Because contact with peers often suffers as a result of the child's parental behaviour, the child cannot gain as much emotional 'reward' anywhere else as at home. Hence, the resistance occurs when the child's responsibilities and the associated affection are 'taken away.'[36]

Gregory Jurkovic

Jurkovic problematises the difficulty of demarcating and defining the concept of parentification.[37] To refine this, he assesses the combination of nine parameters: 1) the manifest presence of protective, caring and responsible behaviour in the child; 2) the content of the obligations that the child has in relation to their role within the family; 3) the scope and duration of these obligations; 4) the person or persons the child has to care for; 5) the age of the child; 6) the extent to which the child internalises their caregiving role, making it part of their personality functioning; 7) the boundaries within the family; 8) the extent to which parentification is common or legitimate within the specific (micro- and macro-cultural) context; and 9) the honesty and fairness that characterise the relationships between family members. Based on these elements, Jurkovic distinguishes between four types of parentification. The first is called destructive parentification. This concerns children or young people with manifestly excessive emotional and/or functional care burdens that are not appropriate for their age. Boundaries are crossed in a way or to an extent that is not appropriate in their cultural context. The tasks assigned to the child are not recognised, supervised, or monitored by the parents and become fundamental to the child/young person's identity.

He refers to a second type as adapted parentification. The care burden for the child is the same as in the previous type, but the child is treated fairly and justly. The child is supported in their task, and the parentification has no decisive influence on their personal development. This type of parentification is often more transient, and relationships normalise once sufficient stability has been restored within the family.

As a third type, Jurkovic proposes healthy (and, in that sense, non-) parentification. The child or young person takes on limited care that is also appropriate to their own level of development. They are helped, recognised, and appreciated by their parents. There is reciprocity and a sense of legitimacy. The necessary boundaries within the family are not crossed.

As a fourth and final variant, Jurkovic mentions infantilisation. The child or young person receives little or no care or responsibility. The parents are excessively accommodating of the child's needs and desires and neglect their own minimal responsibilities.

John Byng-Hall

Parentification leaves its mark on our attachment, among other things. John Byng-Hall is a renowned British therapist who was one of John Bowlby's colleagues and successors at the Tavistock Clinic in London. He is also considered a pioneer of family therapy in Great Britain. He has developed an original body of work based on attachment theories and the structural approach within family therapy, with openings to the intergenerational perspective and the narrative direction. He indeed takes up the views of Minuchin, Boszormenyi-Nagy, and Jurkovic regarding the definition and manifestations of parentification, but adds an attachment dimension to them. He argues that destructive parentification occurs mainly in families with insecure attachment, particularly those of the ambivalent and disorganised type.[38] I quote: 'Insecure attachment patterns in families create fertile ground for parentification, especially when parents lack the internal resources to fulfil their caregiving roles.'[39] In ambivalent attachment, the child feels responsible for the parent's well-being, while in disorganised attachment, the child mainly tries to control chaos and unpredictability. Like Boszormenyi-Nagy, Byng-Hall points to the transgenerational forms that parentification can take. A compulsion to repeat ensures that dysfunctional patterns are passed on from parent to child. Parents who were parentified themselves as children find it difficult to protect their own children emotionally. This can lead to an unconscious transmission of role reversal.

Based on the attachment, the child builds an internal working model of the self and the other, which serves both protective and adaptive functions. Relationships become predictable and safe. If we look at parentification from this theoretical perspective, we see that in the case of pathological parentification, mentalisation fails, both on the part of the parent and on the part of the child. The child, as a functional part of the system, is not thought of as a subject with its own thoughts and feelings, but rather as part of the parent's own functioning. To the extent that the parent, determined by their own history, proves incapable of mentalising the child, the child will also fail to achieve a satisfactory form of mentalisation. Only when the Other thinks of us as a thinking, feeling, and desiring being do we achieve a true psychological/subjective birth. To paraphrase Descartes: she thinks, therefore I am.

Destructive parentification occurs mainly in families with anxious-ambivalent attachment or disorganised attachment. In the first case, overprotectiveness will be an important part of the parenting pattern. When the parent is experiencing stressful factors, the child's closeness is an asset for the parent and a risk for the child, whereby the bond (collusion, symbiosis, etc.) can become too strong. These children exhibit behaviour that is neither age-appropriate nor sufficiently adult. Insecure-disorganised attachment patterns are often associated with a traumatic history in the parents. In this context, children try to take control of their emotional care. Control can translate into caring behaviour on the part of parents, in a begging or bribing manner, or into very punitive, rejecting behaviour. Parentification can also occur in the case of partner conflicts or conflicts due to loss and grief, and can lead to an insecure basis for attachment. Both the security of attachment and mentalising capacity are compromised in destructive parentification. At the same time, working from the perspective of attachment and mentalisation offers a therapeutic opportunity where psychodynamic and contextual thinking can come together. In practice, we find that the so-called pathologically parentified child puts aside their own needs, i.e. their own development, in favour of another goal. And this goal is located elsewhere, Otherways.

Notes

1 Hegel (1830).
2 Santayana (1905, p. 284).
3 Fagan and Durrani (1971).
4 Freud conceived of the Id *(Es)* as the personality's drive system, whereas the unconscious in the narrower sense is essentially a memory system, composed of mnemonic traces of past experiences that guide present behaviour. Two Freud quotations: 'The unconscious contains not only latent memories but also the residues of past experiences' (Freud, 1915, p. 181). 'Memory is present in every psychical system; its function is to store up excitations in a permanent form' (Freud, 1920, p. 18). Laplanche and Pontalis (1973) also make it clear that the *unconscious* is not merely a source of energy (such as the Id), but above all an archive of repressed inscriptions, which implies a memory system.
5 I will leave aside working memory, sensory memory and emotional memory (closely linked to explicit/episodic memory) for the moment.
6 In his *The Interpretation of Dreams* (1900), Freud describes various mechanisms of dream work. These are the psychological processes by which the latent dream material (the unconscious wish content) is transformed into the manifest dream (the story we remember upon waking). Condensation and displacement are the most important, but they are assisted by others. In condensation, multiple latent elements are combined into a single manifest element. For example, people, places or events can merge, often resulting in hybrid or composite figures. The multitude of unconscious associations can also be packaged economically. In displacement, the emotional charge shifts to another element, from foreground to background or vice versa. Other editorial interventions include symbolisation (in which abstract or repressed content is transformed into concrete, often visual symbols) and indirect representation using allusions, metaphors, or analogies. Overdetermination often plays a role, with manifest elements covering several latent ones simultaneously. All of this undergoes final editing or secondary processing, whereby everything is organised (more reasonably) and smoothed out/streamlined/polished.
7 I previously edited a book on parentification (Kinet, 2010).

8 Hetherington (1999).
9 Chen and Panebianco (2019).
10 Kelley et al. (2007).
11 Titzmann (2012).
12 Yew et al. (2017).
13 See the next interlude.
14 Satir (1972, p. 167), Reder et al. (2005, p. 145); Holt (2015, p. 86).
15 Jurkovic (1997, p. 29); Alexander (2014, p. 212).
16 Crittenden (2017, pp. 210–211).
17 Nuttall et al. (2019); Chen and Panebianco (2019).
18 Hooper and Wallace (2010).
19 Byng-Hall (2008); Wang et al. (2017).
20 Hooper (2008).
21 Dayton (2000, p. 63); Love and Robinson (1990).
22 Minuchin et al. (1976, p. 355).
23 Minuchin (1974, pp. 97–98).
24 Chase (1999, p. 8).
25 Minuchin (1981).
26 Wikipedia (n.d.a). 'Salvador Minuchin.' *Wikipedia*. Available at: https://en.wikipedia.org/wiki/Salvador_Minuchin
27 Boszormenyi-Nagy and Spark (1973).
28 Wikipedia (n.d.b). 'Ivan Boszormenyi-Nagy.' *Wikipedia*. Available at: https://en.wikipedia.org/wiki/Ivan_Boszormenyi-Nagy
29 Van der Pas and De Ruiter (1992).
30 Boszormenyi-Nagy and Spark (1973, p. 157).
31 Andolfi (2016).
32 Andolfi et al. (1989).
33 Van der Pas and De Ruiter (ibid.).
34 The term originates from the Norrmalmstorg robbery in Stockholm and the subsequent hostage-taking from 23 to 28 August 1973. The hostages defended their captors, even after the six-day hostage-taking. The criminologist and psychologist Nils Bejerot (1974), who assisted the police at the time, ultimately gave this phenomenon its name.
35 Anna Freud (1936).
36 Van der Pas and De Ruiter (1992, p. 201).
37 Jurkovic (1997); Jurkovic et al. (1999, pp. 93–96).
38 Byng-Hall (1995a, 1995b, 2002).
39 Byng-Hall (2002, p. 378).
40 Hereafter this title is abbreviated to *S. E.*

References

Alexander, P. C. (2014). *Intergenerational Cycles of Trauma and Violence: An Attachment and Family Systems Perspective*, New York: Norton.

Andolfi, M. (2016). *Multigenerational Family Therapy: Tools, Techniques, and Clinical Strategies*. London/New York: Routledge.

Andolfi, M., Angelo, C., and Nichols, M. P. (1989). *Genograms in Family Assessment*. New York: Norton.

Bejerot, N. (1974). *Six Days in August: The Story of the Stockholm Syndrome* (E. King, ed.). New Brunswick, NJ: Rutgers University Press.

Boszormenyi-Nagy, I., and Spark, G. M. (1973). *Invisible Loyalties: Reciprocity in Intergenerational Family Therapy.* New York: Harper and Row, 1984.
Byng-Hall J. (1995a). *Rewriting Family Scripts.* New York: Guilford.
Byng-Hall, J. (1995b). Creating a secure family base: Some implications of attachment theory for family therapy. *Family Process,* 34 (1), 45–58. doi:10.1111/j.1545-5300.1995.00045.x
Byng-Hall, J. (2002). Relieving parentified children's burdens in families with insecure attachment patterns. *Family Process.* 41 (3), 375–388. doi:10.1111/j.1545-5300.2002.41307.x
Byng-Hall, J. (2008). The significance of children fulfilling parental roles: Implications for family therapy. *Journal of Family Therapy,* 30 (2), 147–162. doi:10.1111/j.1467–6427.2008.00423.x
Chase, N. D. (1999). Parentification: An overview of theory, research and societal issues. In: N. D. Chase (ed.), *Burdened Children: Theory, Research and Treatment of Parentification.* Thousand Oaks, CA: Sage.
Chen, C.-Y.-C., and Panebianco, A. (2019). Physical and psychological conditions of parental chronic illness, parentification and adolescent psychological adjustment. *Psychology and Health,* 35 (9), 1075–1094. doi:10.1080/ 08870446.2019.1699091
Crittenden, P. M. (2017). *Raising Parents: Attachment, Representation, and Treatment,* London/New York: Routledge.
Dayton, T. (2000). *Trauma and Addiction: Ending the Cycle of Pain through Emotional Literacy.* Deerfield Beach, FL: Health Communication Inc.
Fagan, B. M., and Durrani, N. (1971). *People of the Earth: An Introduction to World Prehistory.* London/New York: Routledge, 2016.
Freud, A. (1936). The Ego and the Mechanisms of Defence. In *The Writings of Anna Freud* (Vol. II, pp. 3–191). New York: International Universities Press, 1974.
Freud, S. (1900). *The Interpretation of Dreams* (J. Strachey, trans.). New York: Basic Books, 1953.
Freud, S. (1915). The unconscious. In *The Standard Edition of the Complete Psychological Works of Sigmund Freud* (Vol. 14, pp. 159–215). London: Hogarth, 1961.[40]
Freud, S. (1920). Beyond the pleasure principle. In *S. E.* (Vol. 18, pp. 1–64). London: Hogarth, 1961.
Hegel, G. W. F. (1830). *The Philosophy of History* (J. Sibree, trans.). New York: Dover, 1956.
Hetherington, E. M. (1999). Should we stay together for the sake of the children? In E. M. Hetherington (ed.), *Coping with Divorce, Single Parenting, and Remarriage: A Risk and Resiliency Perspective* (pp. 93–116). New York: Lawrence Erlbaum.
Holt, A. (2015). *Working with Adolescent Violence and Abuse Towards Parents: Approaches and Contexts for Intervention.* London/New York: Routledge.
Hooper, L. M. (2008). Defining and understanding Parentification. *The Alabama Counseling Association Journal* 34 (1), 34–43.
Hooper, L. M., and Wallace, S. A. (2010). Evaluating the parentification questionnaire: Psychometric properties and psychopathology correlates. *Contemporary Family Therapy,* 32 (1), 52–68. doi:10.1007/s10591-009-9103-9
Jurkovic, G. J. (1997). *Lost Childhoods: The Plight of the Parentified Child.* New York: Brunner/Mazel, 2014.
Jurkovic, G. J., Morrell, R., Thirkield, A. (1999). Assessing childhood parentification: guidelines for researchers and clinicians. In: N. D. Chase (ed.), *Burdened Children:*

Theory, Research and Treatment of Parentification. London, New Delhi: Sage Publications, 93–96.

Kelley, M. L., French, A., Bountress, K., Keefe, H. A., Schroeder, V., Steer, K., Fals-Stewart, W., and Gumienny, L. (2007). Parentification and family responsibility in the family of origin of adult children of alcoholics. *Addictive Behaviors*, 32 (4), 675–685. doi:10.1016/j.addbeh.2006.06.010

Kinet, M. (ed.) (2010). *Parentificatie. Als het kind te snel ouder wordt*. Antwerpen/Apeldoorn: Garant.

Laplanche, J., and Pontalis, J.-B. (1973). *The Language of Psycho-analysis* (D. Nicholson-Smith, trans.). New York: Norton.

Love, P. and Robinson, P. (1990). *The Emotional Incest Syndrome: What to Do When a Parent's Love Rules Your Life*. New York: Bantam.

Minuchin, S. (1974). *Families and Family Therapy*. Cambridge, MA: Harvard University Press. doi:10.4159/9780674041127

Minuchin, S. (1981). *Family Therapy Techniques*. Cambridge, MA: Harvard University Press.

Minuchin, S. B. Montalvo, B. G. Guerney, B. Rosman, and F. Schumer (1976). *Families of the Slums: An Exploration of Their Structure and Treatment*. New York: Basic Books.

Nuttall, A. K., Zhang, Q., Valentino, K., and Borkowski, J. G. (2019). Intergenerational risk of parentification and infantilization to externalizing moderated by child temperament. *Journal of Marriage and Family*, 81 (3), 648–661. doi:10.1111/jomf.12562

Reder, P., McClure, M., and Jolley, A. (2005). *Family Matters: Interfaces between Child and Adult Mental Health*. London/New York: Routledge.

Santayana, G. (1905). *The Life of Reason: The Phases of Human Progress* (Vol. 1). New York: Scribners.

Satir, V. (1972). *Peoplemaking*. Palo Alto, CA: Science and Behavior Books, 1983.

Titzmann, P. F. (2012). Growing up too soon? Parentification among immigrant and native adolescents in Germany. *Journal of Youth and Adolescence*, 41, 880–893. doi:10.1007/s10964-011-9711-1

Van der Pas, A., and De Ruiter, E. (1992). *Parentificatie: Een contextueel perspectief*. Utrecht: SWP.

Wang, M., Liu, S., and Belsky, J. (2017). Triangulation processes experienced by children in contemporary China. *International Journal of Behavioral Development*, 41 (6), 688–695. doi:10.1177/0165025416662345

Wikipedia (n.d.a). 'Salvador Minuchin.' *Wikipedia*. Available at: https://en.wikipedia.org/wiki/Salvador_Minuchin

Wikipedia (n.d.b). 'Ivan Boszormenyi-Nagy.' *Wikipedia*. Available at: https://en.wikipedia.org/wiki/Ivan_Boszormenyi-Nagy

Yew, S. G. K., Low, W. Y., and Tong, S. F. (2017). The influence of parentification on the well-being of adolescents in Malaysia. *Journal of Family Issues*, 38(13), 1848–1869. doi:10.1177/0192513X15598542

Chapter 4

Intermezzo I

Parentification Cinematic

In this and the following intermezzos, I will illustrate the subject matter clinically. For accessibility and recognisability, I will start with two feature films. The first is *Sorry We Missed You.*[1] It is a social-realist drama (of the kitchen sink genre) by the award-winning director Ken Loach (who has won several awards, including at Cannes). With handheld cameras, a naturalistic dialect and his little-known actors, he immerses you in the Struggle for Life[2] of the ordinary man with this family portrait. The current society, in which we all have to become, as it were, small entrepreneurs of ourselves, is the culprit in the background.

Ricky Turner is a labourer with twelve trades and thirteen accidents to his name. He seizes the opportunity to start working as a parcel courier under his own franchise. Maloney is his tough, no-nonsense boss. To buy the delivery van he needs for the job, Ricky convinces his wife, Abby, to sell their family car. This is despite her initial protests, as she needs the car to work as a home nurse and will now be forced to rely on public transport for her home visits. She was already chronically stressed and underpaid, and her situation is certainly not improved by this. Ricky becomes entangled in a race against time (with Maloney's knife figuratively at his throat). Soon, it all becomes too much for him. He has to constantly rush under time pressure and is fined for the slightest mistake. Their children, Seb and Liza Jane, suffer from the socio-economic situation of their hard-working and therefore unavailable parents. Seb rebels in the form of cheeky defiance, truancy, vandalism, and graffiti. Also, because Abby's ex was physically aggressive, Ricky tries (somewhat too patiently and understandingly) to deal with his son. Liza Jane takes over the caregiving and withdraws. After an argument with his parents, Seb angrily damages all the family portraits hanging in the house. When Ricky cannot find the keys to his van the next morning, he accuses Seb of taking them. Seb denies any involvement and, after a heated exchange, Ricky loses his temper and punches Seb in the face. Both parents are devastated that their children are having such a hard time. Later, Liza Jane confesses that she hid the keys. In her view, all the misery was caused by her father's new job. Back at work, Ricky is brutally mugged while delivering parcels. While he is being treated

DOI: 10.4324/9781003645726-4

for his injuries in the hospital, he receives a call from Maloney informing him that he has to pay a large sum of money because his most important tool (the barcode scanner) was damaged during the mugging. Seb has calmed down and come to his senses. He seeks reconciliation with his parents. Although Ricky has not yet fully recovered, he leaves for work in tears, hurt and distraught, while his wife and two children beg him to stay home and take care of himself.

Although Ken Loach undoubtedly wants to denounce the hidden violence and exploitation of the neoliberal system, he also addresses the damage that children in (not Minuchin's but our contemporary) 'slums' can suffer. Seb rebels in a delinquent manner, but also through artistic street art. Like so many boys, he responds with behavioural disorders (alloplastic). His sister responds autoplastically: she internalises, withdraws emotionally, and takes on a caring role. From a psychoanalytical point of view, parentification plays a role in both her scapegoat and her caring persona. The parents work themselves to the bone to provide their children with sufficient resources, and the latter are forced to take on responsibilities prematurely. The daughter's panic and bedwetting are evidence of the family crisis, while the son's rebelliousness is mainly directed at his father, who tries in vain to maintain his authority. The *Sorry We Missed You* card left at the front door (when the courier is unable to deliver) symbolises the absent parent or their failure. The snowball of parentification starts rolling immediately.

For a narcissistic form of parentification, I refer to *Shine.*[3] The main character in this highly acclaimed blockbuster is David Helfgott. He grows up as a musical prodigy in the suburbs of Adelaide, Australia, but his father, Peter, is very controlling and possessive. During a competition David participates in, it becomes apparent that his father is obsessed with winning. He is strict and ruthless towards David. He demands perfection and does not tolerate any disobedience. David's talent is noticed by a local piano teacher, who takes over his training from his father, Peter. As a teenager, David wins a state competition and is invited by the famous violinist Isaac Stern to continue his studies in the United States. Money is raised and plans are made to make this happen, but ultimately, everything comes to a halt when his father vetoes the idea. He fears that David's departure will damage the family bond. Peter begins to physically and mentally abuse his son, which greatly disturbs the rest of the family. David suffers greatly from his father's approach, but he meets a local novelist who had also co-founded the Australian Communist Party. With her support, David is able and dares to break away from his father and accept the invitation to study music in London. However, his father gives him an ultimatum. If he goes ahead with his plans, he will be banished from the family for good and will never be anyone's son again! When David takes part in a music competition in London, he chooses Rachmaninoff's demanding Third Piano Concerto: a piece he had learned to play as a child so that his father would be proud of him. During his preparatory rehearsals, David becomes extremely nervous. Although he wins the competition, he suffers a mental breakdown and has to be admitted to a psychiatric hospital, where he is even treated with electroconvulsive therapy. The heavy pressure and the problematic relationship with his father have become too much for him. When he has recovered enough to return to Adelaide, his father refuses any reconciliation, and David collapses again. Several years of residential psychiatric treatment follow, after which he is recognised as a former child prodigy by a volunteer there. She takes him home, but there he appears to be more seriously disturbed than she had anticipated. He has difficulty controlling himself, is sometimes unintentionally destructive and needs more care than she can provide. He still finds it difficult to adapt to the outside world. He is noticed again in a restaurant where he sits down at the piano. The owners are amazed by his playing. One of them befriends him and begins to take care of him. In return, David plays the piano there more and more. He meets Gillian, a somewhat eccentric astrologer and restaurant employee. They fall in love and get married. With her support and help, David is able to come to terms with the loss of his father, who has since passed away. A successful comeback concert is organised, heralding the relaunch of his professional musical career. The story, therefore, ends on a hopeful note. Despite traumatic parentification and vulnerability, David finds his way back to both his beloved instrument and to a more or better human connection.

Notes

1 Loach, K. (Director). (2019). *Sorry We Missed You* [Film]. Sixteen Films; Why Not Productions; Wild Bunch.
2 I refer to my next Routledge book: *Psychoanalysis and the Struggle for Love. A Kaleidoscopic View.*
3 Hicks, S. (Director). (1996). *Shine* [Film]. Momentum Pictures.

Chapter 5

Parentification in Various Forms

Role and Function

Parentification is largely a 'normal' phenomenon. Children are very concerned about what is happening with their parents. They are generally much more sensitive than we think, even if they are not (yet) able to express this in words. They also experiment with parental roles, both in their play and in reality. In their play, you often notice how fathers and mothers are portrayed and how roles are creatively adapted. However, the parental role differs from the parental function: a role is defined by convention and is the social translation of what is structurally laid down in the function. The boundaries between the respective roles—child, parent—are guarded, played with, and necessarily crossed in order to maintain them. In psychoanalysis, it is the parental function that is the guarantor, the reference point to which the parental role clings. Freud defines this paternal function in terms of the Oedipus complex. Lacan takes this to a higher level of abstraction with his symbolic order of law, language, and lack. By replacing father and mother with concepts such as the small other and the Big Other, he introduces a terminology applicable regardless of temporal or geographical variants.[1]

What child does not want to grow up and/or become a parent, to be like mummy or daddy? These are, to a large extent, universal desires, in which the child must be lovingly put or kept 'in its place' to establish a right triangle. Parents may delegate certain tasks or functions (temporarily) to their children. However, they do so with sufficient realistic assessment and affective attunement to ensure that the child can effectively bear this responsibility. The child also receives explicit mandate and recognition for their achievements. Under these 'supervised' conditions, it is a learning experience for the child that can rightly be called constructive parentification. After all, the child practises certain skills and/or responsibilities. They slowly and gradually become more mature. This gives them a sense of self-worth and a sense of meaning. If care can be judiciously distributed among family members in this way, there is also more leeway for everyone. The result can be a real win-win situation.

DOI: 10.4324/9781003645726-5

But parentification can also be destructive. For example, the burden on the child may be too heavy or inappropriate for their developmental level. Sometimes the phenomenon is denied or ignored, and the child's real needs are buried beneath it. In this destructive variant, parentification often plays a causal role in psychopathology in adults. It has then caused an imbalance in personality development, leaving a lasting mark on how they relate to others and view the world. In another instance, the child grows up too quickly and/or in leaps and bounds. To this end, they mobilise the necessary strengths and talents. But later on, this begins to 'take its toll' in one way or another and to a greater or lesser extent.

Constructive and Destructive

From the outset, both Boszormenyi-Nagy and Minuchin distinguished between constructive and destructive variants of parentification.[2] Constructive parentification can contribute to responsibility, self-esteem, and competence, provided that tasks are age-appropriate and accompanied by recognition and support. Destructive parentification, on the other hand, jeopardises development by turning the child into an instrument of the parents' unfulfilled needs or traumas. Loyalty becomes pathological: the child loses their childhood and develops patterns that can later lead to depression, anxiety, or relationship difficulties.[3]

The outcome of parentification is moderated by a number of factors, including perception of fairness (if children perceive the caregiving tasks as fair, the consequences are less harmful) and the presence of emotional support (for example, from grandparents or siblings, which can have a buffering effect). The impact of parentification is mediated by perceptions of fairness, an internal locus of control,[4] and attachment style.[5] Positive effects occur mainly when tasks are age-appropriate, emotional support is available,[6] and parents show appreciation for the child's efforts.[7] Cultural views strongly determine how parentification is experienced and assessed.[8] In collectivist cultures, providing care can be interpreted as a form of filial duty, while in individualistic cultures, it is more likely to be seen as transgressive.[9]

Parentification, therefore, requires a sufficiently nuanced perspective. Not every form requires intervention. Instead of problematising the phenomenon by definition, it is important to consider the context, duration, and content of the caregiving role, as well as the child's perception. Prevention of harmful effects can include: consciously assigning age-appropriate care tasks, paying attention to parental appreciation and recognition of the child's efforts, providing guidance on emotional processing and boundaries, and supporting sibling relationships and grandparents. Under certain circumstances, parentification can lead to increased resilience, a sense of responsibility and social competence.[10] Children who feel appreciated in their caregiving role and do not perceive this role as unfair often develop a more positive self-image and better relationships with parents and siblings.[11] Less risky behaviour, such as alcohol consumption or early sexual contact, was also observed.[12]

Adaptive and Pathological

The distinction between constructive and destructive parentification has also been confirmed by later research. Researchers refer to this as adaptive versus pathological parentification.[13] The adaptive form is more temporary or transient. It occurs in a moderate form and aligns with what is culturally normal for the family and the child's developmental level. The child's efforts are also publicly recognised and validated, resulting in fair and encouraging treatment. This form of parentification is more common in girls and can have positive consequences because it promotes empathy and interpersonal skills,[14] fosters adaptive coping, and contributes to self-esteem, psychological maturity, and a motivation for excellence.[15]

Destructive parentification is a prevalent dynamic. In a clinical context, it appears to be one of the causal factors in roughly one-third of adult psychiatric patients.[16] The consequences are wide-ranging: from disruption of attachment[17] to physical impact via stress and immune dysfunction.[18] Psychological boundaries and the child's subjectivity are violated.[19] Through adultification, the child becomes a surrogate partner and is involved in decision-making and finding solutions and/or acts as a friend and confidant,[20] which hinders their own individuation.[21] Most authors point out that parentified children often develop feelings of fear, shame, and guilt, have low self-esteem, are distrustful in relationships, and exhibit more or less serious depressive tendencies.[22] Parentification in childhood appears to be a decisive factor in an adult's later relational style.[23] They invariably take on a caring role towards other adults and develop a personality that revolves around care and service. We find in them what John Bowlby calls 'compulsive giving.'[24]

Two very comprehensive overview publications on the advantages and disadvantages of parentification have recently been published. Jacinda Dariotis and colleagues base their findings on a systematic literature review,[25] while Ruziana Masiran and colleagues base theirs on an integrated narrative review.[26] This overview also shows that parentification need not be negative. Positive outcomes include: improved parent-child relationships, especially in moderate forms of emotional parentification; stronger bonds with siblings, particularly when caregiving tasks are focused on brothers or sisters; increased resilience, responsibility, and self-esteem, especially when parentification is accompanied by parental recognition and appreciation; and better social adjustment and school performance, particularly in families where children feel valued in their caregiving role. A prerequisite for these positive effects is that the role assignment is age-appropriate, recognised and supported by the parents, and that the child experiences the situation as fair and meaningful.

At the same time, several studies confirm the potential harmfulness of parentification, especially in the case of prolonged and emotionally charged role reversals. Possible negative effects include: psychological complaints, such as depression, anxiety, reduced self-esteem and impostor syndrome; disrupted attachment and intimate relationships, especially in girls who become emotionally involved in parental problems; limited emotional expression and self-regulation, as children learn to suppress their own feelings in favour of others; and intergenerational transmission. In the latter case, parentification leads to a less warm upbringing by the next generation. Prolonged or emotionally charged parentification is associated with depression,[27] anxiety, low self-esteem,[28] impaired attachment,[29] and disruption of intimate relationships,[30] as well as an increased risk of externalising behaviour in the next generation.[31]

Various Forms

We note that Boszormenyi-Nagy defines the parentified position in various ways. He refers to the abused child and the highly idealised child (who will ultimately be unable to fulfil their role anyway). There is the child in the role of scapegoat, caught between conflicting loyalties, taking on a mediating role, for example, in a conflictual parental relationship. There is the caring child, the child who is kept small, or the child who is not given any boundaries by the adult.[32] Boszormenyi-Nagy places loyalty alongside attachment. Loyalty is grafted onto the relationship, while attachment is more of an intrapsychic counterpart. The loyalty in question concerns unconscious, internalised obligations and expectations that connect the child to their family of origin, sometimes even across several generations. It is invisible but can be decisive for the decisions, relationships, and identity of the person concerned. It is a kind of ethical and moral ledger that keeps track of what has been given and received in terms of love and care or, conversely, neglect and harm. When the balance is disturbed, invisible loyalties can 'take revenge' in unreasonable (e.g. towards 'innocent' others) and/or self-destructive ways. The child remains (unconsciously) loyal to a parental figure, even when that figure was abusive or absent. This 'loyalty' can take various forms. For example, the child may repeat the same pattern as the parent, sabotage themselves, engage in a pattern of caring relationships, or form other dysfunctional relationships. More specifically, in the case of parentification, a deep loyalty plays a role, for example, towards an emotionally overwhelmed, unavailable, and/or traumatised parent figure. Out of a sense of justice, love, or duty, the child intuitively wants to fill the parental gaps. A pattern of parentification can be passed on transgenerationally. The child is seen as a source of emotional support or as a means of compensating for unmet needs. The parentified child develops symptoms of anxiety and depression in which guilt plays an important role. When it tries to break free, it feels as if it is abandoning or betraying the distressed parent. From a therapeutic perspective, Boszormenyi-Nagy believes it is important to make the child aware of the dynamics described above. The aim is to enable the child to free themselves from unjustified feelings of responsibility or guilt and to prioritise their own needs and boundaries.

Achieving a more just relationship through insight is the most important therapeutic task in all of this: modifying destructive parentification into recognition and validation. In other words, recognising and acknowledging the care that the child provides and restoring responsibilities. Deparentification is not only a process for the child; the parentifying parent also plays a role. For psychoanalysts, however, the question arises as to whether (especially cognitive) awareness is sufficient to simply correct 'wrong' feelings and behaviours that have become established.

Too Close

When we look at the concept of parentification in the literature, we encounter all kinds of closely related terms, such as adultification or spousification, boundary dissolution, role reversal, emotional incest, little parents, or young carers.[33] Some family therapists consider emotional parentification to be a form of emotional or '*covert*' (hidden form of) incest. This covert incest would occur when the child becomes the primary object of the parent's affection, love, passion, and concerns. Out of the emptiness and loneliness of a prolonged, unhappy relationship, the parent turns to the child as a kind of surrogate partner. In such a configuration, the child may feel trapped and used, just as in overt incest. When the child wants to regain his autonomy, play, or make friends, he feels guilty and lonely because these desires make him feel guilty. Therefore, he renounces these desires in order to devote himself entirely to the parent. This is a psychological marriage, and there is a danger that a kind of electricity will develop within the parent-child relationship without actual sexual acts taking place. Patricia Love refers to this as the 'chosen child'. Boundaries are lost, and both 'partners' become enmeshed with each other. I will return to this later.

Over time, Boszormenyi-Nagy began to associate the (contextual) concept of parentification with the (psychoanalytical) concept of projective identification. Parents project split-off needs onto their children, cling possessively to their child, or derive benefits from them.[34] The child cannot ward off the projection, and the positions persist, leading to a pathological constellation. Fundamental to pathological parentification is not only the role reversal but also the breach of trust. Parentification occurs when the asymmetry of the relationship is not respected: needs are delegated, and the child is unfairly blamed or given responsibility but not recognition. This makes the child 'destructively entitled'. As the one who pays the price, the child wants to seek redress for the injustice done to them and, sooner or later, make the Other pay (also in the transference and therefore when it is not the basis of the injustice).

Later, family therapists also link parentification to the concept of projective identification, thus further bridging the gap to psychoanalysis. Projective identification is understood to mean the projection of split-off parts of the personality onto another person. They are, as it were, downloaded onto the other person, who is thereby so strongly influenced in the interaction that they increasingly behave in accordance with the projection. According to Heinrich Racker, we can further divide this mechanism into the concordant and complementary forms.[35] Applied to the therapeutic encounter, in the concordant form, a part of the self ends up with the therapist. The latter identifies, for example, with the patient's unrecognised child part. It strives to please the parents, and the therapist or the parentified child unconsciously starts to behave in the same way. In the complementary form, on the other hand, an inner object ends up with the therapist. The therapist catches himself, for example, acting in a counter-transference manner, treating the helpless patient in a haughty, mocking way, just as the child, without really wanting to, treats his parent like the devil. In other words, in projective identification, the intrapsychic spills over into the interpersonal. Emotionally speaking, parts of oneself end up with the other and parts of the other end up with oneself. It is a mechanism from early development, when no clear boundary has yet been established between I and Thou. The Lacanian mirror stage and the imaginary register (more on this later) are at the forefront. Technically speaking, self-object differentiation is still unstable. Arthur Rimbaud's expression applies here in both directions: *Je est un autre.* I am another, and the other is I. In a constant oscillation between mirroring and marking by the parents, the basic security and mentalising capacity necessary for the small child are built up during this early period, if all goes well.

Further Typology

Walter Oppenoorth describes two forms of helper parenting in this context.[36] In the first form, the parentified child undergoes a forced development towards independence. The child performs tasks far beyond their age level, usually in the caring sphere, with siblings and/or parents. This is at the expense of their own developmental tasks, such as peer contact and emotional development. In the second form, the child undergoes delayed development and remains extremely dependent under the influence of the parental need to continue caring for the child. Since these are two clearly different expressions of the same phenomenon, Oppenoorth refers to active and passive helper parenting, respectively. In his description of parentification, Oppenoorth emphasises the role of the parents, from which the loyal child cannot escape. According to him, the mechanism of projective identification in the parents underlies parentification. The impact of this parental defence mechanism on the child is enormous. The child increasingly conforms to the split-off part of the parent. This reinforces the parent's primitive defence mechanism. The result is a vicious circle of mutual dependence. When the child breaks the bond with the parent in adulthood, often abruptly, it carries within it a complementary interaction pattern that can repeat itself 'fatally' (e.g. transgenerationally).[37] Frans Van Mierlo and colleagues elaborate on the importance of projective identification in the process of parentification.[38] The different forms of parentification vary depending on which part of themselves the parent projects onto the child, as well as on the (psychoanalytically understandable) theme in which the parent is stuck. There are two poles on the continuum: the child must satisfy oral care needs or must satisfy the narcissistic behavioural expectations of the parent(s).

In the first (most 'classical') case, everything revolves around the oral theme of care between parent and child. Within this, there are two further possibilities. The parentification of the caring child (Oppenoorth's active parentification) is most easily recognised. Caring children take on household tasks, provide emotional support and comfort to parents and siblings, and are often their first and only conversation partner and confidant. These children are called 'angels': they are sweet, accommodating, and helpful. From a very early age, they have developed a sensitivity to empathise with their parents and try to meet their needs. They implicitly sense the pain of unresolved issues from their parents' past and will try to heal or alleviate this pain. The parents have often had a severe lack of parental care and are overburdened and unavailable to their children. The caring child will try to fill this void. The caring child has little contact with their peers because there is always something to do at home. They prefer the company of older children or adults. They always use their 'common sense,' and their mentalising ability is mainly focused on others' needs. This great capacity for empathy is accompanied by a poignant lack of awareness of their own needs and desires. The child also lacks playfulness, spontaneity, and exuberance. They imagine themselves to be strong and believe that they must not be weak. They find it difficult to recognise and communicate their own needs, wishes, and feelings. They can only give and find it difficult to receive help or attention without feeling that the other person is being short-changed or given too much. Because caring for their parents rarely helps, children often feel guilty and incompetent. Feelings of inferiority and a negative self-image are the result. In adulthood, exhaustion and depressive symptoms may develop. After all, they become entangled in a relationship pattern in which others parasitise them.

A more subtle form of parentification occurs when the child (for the caring parent) has to remain a child, as it were. Often, the youngest children are most affected by this. This infantilising 'keeping small' (however loving and well-intentioned) is detrimental to individuation and sexualisation. All responsibilities are permanently borne by the parents. The child grows up distorted. They continue to expect others to give them what they need without having to do anything themselves. The laws of social interaction (symmetrical relationships and reciprocity) are not established. These children feel cheated and deprived. Their frustration tolerance is low. They cannot handle being told no. Feelings of omnipotence, boundlessness, difficulty with hierarchy, difficulty tolerating criticism, and manipulative behaviour are characteristic of this indulgent form of parentification.

On the other hand, the child can also become parentified due to a narcissistic theme. They become stuck in (behavioural) expectations because of the parent(s). As in *Shine's* example, this may involve certain narcissistic frustrations of the parents that leave a compelling mark on the child. But the scapegoat phenomenon can also be considered a form of parentification. The child is unfairly forced to take responsibility for another's burdens or transgressions.

A scapegoat arises in a family with major tensions, usually between the parents. The child acts as a lightning rod to retain some control over the situation. Psychoanalysts recognise such small wars as a schizoid-paranoid constellation. The phenomenon is characterised by insecurity, action, and the hegemony of primitive defence mechanisms such as denial, splitting, projective identification, and omnipotent control. The child takes on the blame for the tensions as a scapegoat. It sacrifices itself and is sacrificed for the family's benefit. This leads to a damaged self-image, feelings of inferiority, jealousy, and/or distrust of others: an obvious breeding ground for all kinds of personality disorders.

The Experience of Parentification

The following are typical statements from adults who developed a pattern of parentification as children:

- 'My mother complained a lot about the emotional abuse she suffered at the hands of her parents and about her sexual abuse. I tried to appease my father as much as possible so that he wouldn't lash out verbally or physically at my younger brothers. If I hadn't kept some order and regularity in our home, it would have been constant chaos and crisis.'
- 'Every time my father cheated on her, I had to comfort my mother.'
- 'My father took me to his mistresses and I had to keep his secrets.'

A 'pattern,' because there is no emotional parentification in one-off incidents where a parent is upset and finds comfort in one of the children. It is a persistent role reversal in which the child has to 'serve' to satisfy various emotional needs. The child learns that they must grow up quickly and set aside their own social and emotional agenda to maintain peace and balance at home for their parent(s). They are well-behaved, easy-going, capable, and sensible children who perform well. There are apparently no problems to be noticed or seen in them. As children, they are little adults, but as adults, sooner or later, an unpleasant surprise emerges: in a way that is 'incomprehensible' (to themselves and those around them), they feel or behave like small children.

Shirley Schorr and her colleagues conducted semi-structured interviews with adult participants who retrospectively described their experiences of parentification.[39] They used a qualitative method that focuses on the subjective meanings that individuals attach to their experiences.[40] The method allows both explicit themes and implicit affective structures to be articulated. The most important metaphor that emerges is walking on eggshells: 'Like stepping on glass.' It is a metaphor that is frequently used by the respondents. It aptly illustrates how cautious, fearful, and painful it is to move within a parentifying context and how little room there is for relaxation or spontaneity. The image also reflects continuous hypervigilance and a lack of basic security. Five central themes recur in the emotional experience of parentification. First, emotional confusion. 'I couldn't tell where I ended and they began.' Parentification entails a fundamental disruption of the self-other boundary. The child's caring position leads to diffuse boundaries, making it difficult to distinguish their own needs from those of the parent. This confusion is not only cognitive, but also affective: the child internalises the parent's pain and needs as if they were their own. This aligns with Donald Winnicott's description of the danger of a false self, arising when the child's true self is not reflected.[41] Peter Fonagy and his colleagues also point out that the absence of marked mirroring leads to a deficient mentalising capacity.[42] The second core experience is hypervigilance and anxiety: 'I was always bracing for impact.' Children in parentifying families develop chronic hypervigilance. They constantly anticipate their parents' emotional states to protect themselves and others. This excessive vigilance is often accompanied by fear of outbursts, rejection, or blame. The child becomes an emotional thermometer for the family or a canary in the coal mine. This psychodynamic shows parallels with the concept of 'affective contagion' in children of depressed mothers.[43] It was also found in Sándor Ferenczi's description of children who dissociatively adapt to the needs of their parent(s).[44] Thirdly, there are the inner conflicts and moral dissonance. 'I felt guilty for being angry.' The experience of parentification is often associated with ambivalence: the child feels obliged to be caring and loyal, but also experiences anger and frustration. However, this anger is often internalised as guilt or shame. The respondent feels bad or ungrateful when he or she allows negative feelings towards the parents.

A communication system develops in which any expression of autonomy is interpreted as betrayal or a lack of loyalty. This internal contradiction can lead to chronic depression or perfectionism as a result of an excessively strict conscience. The fourth element is a disruption of identity development and a lost childhood. 'I never got to be a kid.' Children who end up in a parental role often have a distorted perception of their childhood and have felt old or responsible since their earliest memories. They have a lot of mileage on the clock and are tired or burnt out after long hours and hard work. Many continue to seek identification in caring roles (such as in their profession or choice of partner) even in adulthood. In Lacanian (or Bionian) terms, we can speak here of a fixation of the subject on the fantasy of the Other: the child becomes the mirror/container of the Other's desires/needs and lacks its own position in the symbolic. Ultimately, there is a paradoxical feeling of both strength and loss. 'It made me who I am, for better or worse.' Many respondents also recognise their parentification as a source of resilience, empathy, and competence. They feel that their experiences have made them mature, and they often develop a strong sense of responsibility. At the same time, they recognise that this growth process took place at the expense of their subjective integrity.

Psychoanalytical?

We will discuss further on that it is mainly psychoanalysts who expose the intrapsychic, if not phantasmatic, roots of parentification in the child's mind. Is it called upon or does it feel called upon? They also remind us that this can happen in a completely hidden and/or invisible way. Moreover, it can nevertheless become embedded as a deep and persistent template in adult psychosocial life. This template repeats itself through transference and repetition compulsion across various relationships and areas of life, and must be analysed again and again according to the motto 'to dissect is to die.' In other words, Freud's well-known ironic metaphor about trauma counselling is certainly also applicable to parentified adults.[45] If a house burns down because of an overturned oil lamp, it is unfortunately not enough to simply put the lamp back upright. Instead, all damage must be assessed to ensure the construction of a new (and preferably fire-safe) home. This requires a psychoanalytical investigation into the furthest corners of the psyche and a great deal of remembering, repeating, and working through to get parentification 'out of your system.' Now that the term 'system' has been mentioned, I would like to emphasise the following from the outset. Especially in the case of children or young people still living at home, the treatment of parentification requires a minimum integration of a systemic and a psychoanalytical perspective.[46]

The literature on parentification is mainly situated in interactional and contextual regions. It concerns processes that occur in the realm of behavioural reality, whether or not they are based on unconscious factors. Parentification also appears (despite its circular nature) predominantly as a process originating with the parents. Parentification emerges as a process actively induced by parents in their child, enacted through their actual interactions. For example, it is said that in parentification, parents project split-off needs and/or personality traits onto their child, influencing the child's interactions in ways that increasingly conform to the split-off parental part. Out of natural loyalty, the child adapts to the parental conscious and unconscious needs. Even from a psychoanalytical perspective, it is sometimes described in these terms. Han Blankstein describes parentification as follows: 'The child is placed by the parent in a parental role in relation to themselves.'[47] Apparently, from this perspective, parentification clearly and unilaterally originates from the parent. To put it bluntly: the parents are the perpetrators, the child is the victim. Parents parentify, children *are* parentified.[48] Typically psychoanalytically, however, a central role is assigned to unconscious, phantasmatic, and internal processes (also in parentification). She finds an approach that is based exclusively or predominantly on the relational dynamics at the level of behavioural reality to be insufficient. Secondly, she also zooms in more on the child as an active agent in the process of parentification. After all, projective identification also plays a role *in* the parent and *because of* the child. For example, the child can split off the dependence he hates and project it onto the parent, making him appear more independent. Or the child has an unconscious desire to take the parent's place. Melanie Klein puts it as follows: 'The unconscious minds of the children very often correspond to the mother's unconscious mind.'[49] Donald Winnicott pointed out the danger of a false self that arises when the child lives in response to the needs of others.[50] For Lacan, parentification is an extension of a lack of paternal function: the child is not protected from the incestuous proximity of the Other and remains locked in a kind of false idyll.[51]

Psychoanalysis and Destructive Parentification

Various psychoanalytic theories discuss the consequences of destructive parentification. Examples include attachment theory,[52] object relations theory,[53] and self-psychology.[54] According to attachment theory, there are consistent positive correlations between parental warmth, sensitivity, and responsiveness and a healthy socio-emotional life later on. When children are forced to care for parents or siblings to satisfy their need for attachment, parentified children internalise negative representations of themselves and others, thereby perpetuating transgenerational parentification.[55] On the one hand, adults who were parentified as children will continue to play that caring role in their relationships, while on the other hand, they will focus on their own deficiencies in their children in order to obtain emotional nourishment from them and satisfy their narcissistic or relational needs.[56]

According to object relations theories, parentification can instil a 'fear of breakdown' in the child.[57] This refers to an unthinkable state of mind rooted in the mother's inability to care for her child adequately, causing the child to defensively split their psyche. It internalises the parent's ego ideal and is forced to renounce its own desires, needs, or goals to satisfy the parent's unfulfilled needs. Similarly, self-psychology states that a cohesive self can only be achieved if the child's own narcissistic needs (mirroring of greatness, idealisation of the parent, experiencing a soulmate connection with the parent) are sufficiently satisfied by the parent(s). If this is not the case, a fragile self develops, lacking coherence and sufficient, consistent self-esteem and self-worth.[58] In this model, both the need to emotionally care for the parental figure and to bow to their hostile and/or manipulative control ensure that the parentified person develops either a masochistic-tinged narcissistic vulnerability,[59] or a blatant narcissistic personality disorder in adulthood.[60] In any case, unmet parental needs can foster a sense of inferiority, seriously hindering the development of an autonomous and robust self.[61]

The Unconscious and the Big Other

The Big Other is reflected in our unconscious. What we do or do not like seems natural, but is (without us realising it) largely culturally determined. Both the microculture of family and the macroculture of the spirit of the times leave their mark on our lives. Social changes undoubtedly increase vulnerability to parentification. In our time, we are witnessing, among other things, a steady erosion of the traditional family. As a result, children are a lot freer and often more detached. At the same time, they find less protection from all kinds of stimuli. David Elkind talks about *The Hurried Child*;[62] most recognisable in his modern classic is the digital acceleration in which the internet and social media increase the pressure. Children are exposed to adult themes such as sexuality, violence, and consumerism, and a (competitive) battle of all against all is instilled. There is little room left for rest or seclusion. Children are also approached as consumers from an early age. They are bombarded with products that push them towards adulthood, such as fashion or beauty ideals. Or they have an overloaded schedule that leaves little time for free play or for just *being themselves* instead of *acting* extraordinary. At first, children eagerly take on all these 'challenges,' but this gives them a misleading illusion of maturity. At the same time, these children still need their parents to care for, watch over, and protect them. In fact, nowadays there is an increasingly long period of dependence (necessary) in order for them to develop sufficiently into independent adults.

Children and Adults

Children are little helpers. Unhindered by any experience or knowledge, they can easily lose themselves in the maelstrom of parentification. In the case of children who are still growing up and living at home, all those involved need to respond to this often overlooked and insidious psychodynamic in a timely and mentalising manner. Both the family and the child deserve a separate approach in this regard. In adult patients, the mechanism of parentification has often already left a clear mark on their relationship with the Big Other. By analogy with cancer treatment or trauma counselling, not only the tumour but also the proverbial metastases must be thoroughly addressed.

From a therapeutic perspective, this has several 'logical' consequences. Parentification first requires recognition and validation of the care provided, combined with the restoration of generational boundaries. The therapeutic space must function as a holding environment, in which regression, mourning, and separation are possible.[63] The treatment aims to restore the distinction between one's own feelings and needs and those of others, and to give the child—or the adult who once was a child—the chance to truly be a child.[64] This immediately highlights a difference between parentified children and parentified adults. With children, the main aim is to modify destructive parentification through recognition and validation of it. The care the child provides must be recognised and acknowledged to restore legitimate responsibilities. De-parentification is, of course, not only a process for the child; the parentifying parent(s) also have a role to play. For psychoanalysts, however, the question arises as to whether (mainly cognitive) awareness is sufficient to simply correct 'wrong' feelings and behaviours that have become established in the meantime.

The long-term effects of destructive parentification are both deeply ingrained and spread throughout the adult's psyche. These include chronic feelings of guilt and difficulty maintaining and guarding boundaries, difficulty receiving care and/or trusting others, hyper-empathy and excessive identification with the pain of others (typical statement: 'I feel like a sponge'), separation anxiety and compulsive caring, identity diffusion, and difficulty accessing one's true desires and needs.

First Conclusion

Parentification lies at the intersection of system and psyche, loyalty and identity, vulnerability and strength. It is a transgenerational phenomenon that leaves deep scars in attachment, subjectivity and interpersonal relationships. It requires a nuanced approach in which destructive forms are recognised and addressed promptly, while constructive variants are recognised as sources of growth.

Parentification is an important risk factor for the development of all kinds of psychopathology. It can have a disastrous impact on attachment and/or determine, if not mortgage, later relationships with others. The child is called upon and/or feels called upon to take on certain inappropriate responsibilities. It may also presume to do so. In this way, it grows up too quickly, as it were. In doing so, it mobilises the necessary strengths and talents. However, in later life, this phenomenon can have various repercussions. As is well known, the quality of attachment is one of the most important determinants of all pathology (not only psychological but also physical). The quality of attachment not only calibrates our resilience[65] but also our immune system.[66] The relevance of parentification for mental and other health can therefore hardly be overestimated.

In this introduction, I have explained the more contextual or systemic mechanisms of parentification rather than the psychodynamic ones. In short, I considered parentification to be an extremely relevant and prevalent phenomenon. From a psychoanalytical perspective, I discussed the false self and the false idyll. Both are, of course, entirely *sincere* phenomena. In all cases of parentification, the third party's failure will also be evident. The paternal function that should protect the child from the essentially incestuous nature of emotional abuse falls short. As a result, the child is left with a difficult calling:

trying to fill the 'gap' in or of the early Big Other.[67] There is no third party who, so to speak, puts a stop (the phallus) to the deadly combination of lust and displeasure that this causes those involved.[68] The Oedipal triangle contains more curves than straight lines, and according to the Lacanians, this structural configuration plays a decisive role in processes of parentification. The child must 'serve' (financially, instrumentally, emotionally, socially, and/or sexually) for something for which it does not actually serve.

Some form or degree of parentification is ubiquitous among children of parents with alcohol dependence. Moreover, it affects not only patients but also many care providers. The following chapters focus on what parental alcoholism means for the development of their children. Therapists often come from parentified families themselves and, to a greater or lesser extent, correspond to the figure of the wounded healer. Their calling can be understood both as a symptom of unresolved problems or conflicts and as a source of motivation to perform healing work.[69] This second subgroup of parentification will be discussed in more detail later on.

Notes

1 Lacan distinguishes between the small other and the Big Other. The little other is the imaginary other—the mirror image, the equal, the rival, someone with whom we identify or to whom we attach ourselves. The Big Other is, on the one hand, the other in his radical otherness and, on the other hand, the symbolic Other—who represents the place of language, law, boundary, authority, lack, difference, and desire. In psychoanalytic therapy, it is the symbolic Other (as a structure rather than a person) where presumed knowledge is located. For a concise Lacanian introduction see Bailly (2012) or Kinet (2024, pp. 106–133).
2 Boszormenyi-Nagy and Spark (1973), Minuchin (1971, 1981).
3 Fonagy et al. (1994); Hooper et al. (2011).
4 Williams and Francis (2010).
5 Baggett et al. (2015).
6 Napora (2016).
7 Thastum et al. (2008).
8 Cho and Lee (2019); Shin and Hecht (2013).
9 Jackson et al. (2016).
10 Stein et al. (2015); Gilford and Reynolds (2011).
11 Borchet et al. (2020); Tompkins (2007).
12 Sang et al. (2014); Shin and Hecht (2013).
13 Byng-Hall (2008); Saha (2016).
14 Champion et al. (2009).
15 Byng-Hall (2008).
16 Kinet (2008).
17 Madden and Shaffer (2016).
18 de Kloet (2009).
19 Nuttall et al. (2019).
20 Garber (2011).
21 Goldner et al. (2021); Macfie, Brumariu and Lyons-Ruth (2015).
22 Jurkovic (1997), Byng-Hall (2008).
23 Valleau et al. (1995).

24 Bowlby (1980).
25 Dariotis et al. (2023).
26 Masiran et al. (2023). They studied 61 articles selected from Scopus, PubMed, Google Scholar, and other sources.
27 Cho and Lee (2019).
28 Black and Sleigh (2013).
29 Madden and Shaffer (2016).
30 Baggett et al. (2015).
31 Van Loon et al. (2017).
32 Onderwaater (2009).
33 Burton (2007), Macfie, Brumariu, and Lyons-Ruth (2015); Kerig (2005); Love and Robinson (1990), Byng-Hall (2008); Aldridge and Becker (1993).
34 Boszormenyi-Nagy and Krasner (1986).
35 Racker (1968).
36 Oppenoorth (1990, 1994).
37 Oppenoorth (1990, pp. 32, 33).
38 Van Mierlo et al. (1998).
39 Schorr and Goldner (2023).
40 Interpretative Phenomenological Analysis (IPA) by Smith et al. (2009).
41 Winnicott (1965).
42 Fonagy et al. (2002).
43 Lyons-Ruth et al. (2006).
44 Ferenczi (1932).
45 Freud (1917, p. 451) 'Probably not more than if the fire brigade, called to deal with a house that had been set on fire by an overturned oil lamp, contented themselves with removing the lamp from the room in which the blaze had started.'
46 Kinet (2008).
47 Blankstein (1970, p. 190).
48 Thys (2010).
49 Klein (1937, p. 320).
50 Winnicott (1965).
51 Lacan (1966).
52 Bowlby (1980).
53 Winnicott (1965).
54 Kohut (1971).
55 Hooper (2008).
56 Engelhardt (2012).
57 Winnicott (1965, 1974).
58 Kohut (1971).
59 Nehrig et al. (2019); Van Buren and Meehan (2015).
60 Taillieu et al. (2016).
61 Goldner, Sachar, and Abir (2019); Goldner et al. (2021).
62 Elkind (1981).
63 Winnicott (1965).
64 Fonagy et al. (2002).
65 Fonagy et al. (1994).
66 de Kloet (2009, p. 547).
67 For clarity's sake, this can be any significant parental figure.
68 Lacan calls this painful 'enjoyment' '*jouissance*,' which (as will be explained later) literally means 'usufruct.' We will suffice here to refer to Verhaeghe (2009, p. 15), who calls this *jouissance* 'a difficult concept' in a footnote: 'It is what we experience in the borderland between lustful, controllable tension and what lies *beyond* it,

with the result that we lose 'ourselves' (read: our sense of identity). For Lacan, moreover, this experience is inexpressible, which does not make it any easier to define. How does libido 'feel'? A precarious surfing on the wave of desire? I have previously devoted a great deal of (neuro)psychoanalytical attention to jouissance (Kinet, 2023).

69 Winer (1994); Gabbard (1995).

References

Aldridge, J. S. and Becker, S. (1993). *Children Who Care: Inside the World of Young Carers.* Loughborough: Loughborough University.

Baggett, E., Shaffer, A., and Muetzelfeld, H. (2015). Father-daughter parentification and young adult romantic relationships among college women. *Journal of Family Issues*, 36 (6), 760–783. doi:10.1177/0192513X13499759

Bailly, L. (2012). *Lacan: A Beginner's Guide.* New York: Simon and Schuster.

Black, K., and Sleigh, M. J. (2013). The impact of parentification on the adjustment of young adults. *Child Psychiatry and Human Development*, 44 (5), 676–688.

Blankstein, J. H. (1970). Gezinstherapie, vanuit psychoanalytisch gezichtspunt. *Tijdschrift voor Psychiatrie*, 12, 186–197.

Borchet, J., Lewandowska-Walter, A., Połomski, P., Peplinska, A., and Hooper, L. M. (2020). We are in this together: Retrospective parentification, sibling relationships, and self-esteem. *Journal of Child and Family Studies*, 2982–2991. doi:10.1007/s10826–10020–01723–01723

Boszormenyi-Nagy, I., and Spark, G. M. (1973). *Invisible loyalties: Reciprocity in intergenerational family therapy.* New York: Harper & Row, 1994.

Boszormenyi-Nagy, I., and Krasner, B. R. (1986). *Between Give and Take: A Clinical Guide to Contextual Therapy.* New York: Brunner/Mazel.

Bowlby, J. (1980). *Attachment and Loss: Vol. 3. Loss: Sadness and Depression.* New York: Basic Books.

Burton, L. (2007). Childhood adultification in economically disadvantaged families: A conceptual model. *Family Relations*, 56 (4), 329–345. doi:10.1111/j.1741–3729.2007.00463.x

Byng-Hall, J. (2008). The significance of children fulfilling parental roles: Implications for family therapy. *Journal of Family Therapy*, 30 (2), 147–162. doi:10.1111/j.1467–6427.2008.00423.x

Champion, J. E., Jaser, S. S., Reeslund, K. L., Simmons, L., Potts, J. E., Shears, A. R., and Compas, B. E. (2009). Caretaking behaviors by adolescent children of mothers with and without a history of depression. *Journal of Family Psychology*, 23 (2), 156–166. doi:10.1037/a0014978

Cho, A. R., and Lee, S. Y. (2019). Exploring effects of childhood parentification on adult-depressive symptoms in Korean college students. *Journal of Clinical Psychology*, 75 (4), 801–813. doi:10.1002/jclp.22737

Dariotis, J. K., Lorenzo, K., Turkheimer, E., Perlstein, M. B., and White, C. N. (2023). Parentification: Vulnerability, reactivity, resilience, and thriving—A mixed-methods systematic literature review. *Adversity and Resilience Science*, 4 (2), 127–166.

De Kloet, E. R. (2009). Stress: neurobiologisch perspectief. *Tijdschrift voor Psychiatrie*, 51 (8), 541–550.

Elkind, D. (1981). *The Hurried Child: Growing Up Too Fast Too Soon* (3rd edn). Cambridge, MA: Da Capo Press, 2007.

Engelhardt, J. A. (2012). The developmental implications of parentification: Effects on childhood attachment. *Graduate Student Journal of Psychology*, 14, 45–52.

Ferenczi, S. (1932). *The Clinical Diary of Sándor Ferenczi* (M. Balint, ed.; M. Dupont, trans.). Cambridge, MA: Harvard University Press, 1988.

Fonagy, P., Steele, M., Steele, H., Higgitt, A. and Target, M. (1994). The theory and practice of resilience. *Journal of Child Psychology and Psychiatry*, 15, 231–257.

Fonagy, P., Gergely, G., Jurist, E., and Target, M. (2002). *Affect Regulation, Mentalization, and the Development of the Self.* New York: Other Press.

Freud, S. (1917). Introductory lectures on psycho-analysis (Part III). In *S.E.* (Vol. 16, pp. 243–463). London: Hogarth, 1963.

Gabbard, G. O. (1995). When the patient is a therapist. Special challenges in the psychoanalysis of mental health professionals. *Psychoanalytic Review*, 82, pp. 709–725.

Garber, B. D. (2011). Parental alienation and the dynamics of the enmeshed parent–child dyad: Adultification, parentification, and infantilization. *Family Court Review*, 49 (2), 322–335. doi:10.1111/j.1744-1617.2011.01374.x

Gilford, T. T., and Reynolds, A. (2011). 'My mother's keeper': The effects of parentification on black female college students. *Journal of Black Psychology*, 37 (1), 55–77. doi:10.1177/0095798410372624

Goldner, L., Sachar, S. C., and Abir, A. (2019). Mother-adolescent parentification, enmeshment and adolescents' intimacy: The mediating role of rejection sensitivity. *Journal of Child and Family Studies*, 28 (1), 192–201. doi:10.1007/ s10826–10018–1244–1248

Goldner, L., Jakobi, C. D., Schorr, S., Dakak, S., and Shawahne, N. (2021). Keep it quiet: Mother–daughter parentification and difficulties in separation–individuation shaping daughters' authentic/true self and self-silencing: A mediation model. *Psychoanalytic Psychology*, 39 (2), 165–174. doi:10.1037/pap0000352

Hooper, L. M. (2008) Defining and understanding parentification. *The Alabama Counseling Association Journal* 34 (1), 34–43.

Hooper, L. M., DeCoster, J., White, N., and Voltz, M. L. (2011). Characterizing the magnitude of the relation between self-reported childhood parentification and adult psychopathology: A meta-analysis. *Journal of Clinical Psychology*, 67 (10), 1028–1043. doi:10.1002/jclp.20807

Jackson, E. F., Raval, V. V., Bendikas-King, E. A., Raval, P. H., and Trivedi, S. S. (2016). Cultural variation in reports of subjective experience of parent-child boundary dissolution among emerging adults. *Journal of Family Issues*, 37 (5), 671–691. doi:10.1177/0192513X15576280

Jurkovic, G. J. (1997). *Lost Childhoods: The Plight of the Parentified Child.* New York: Brunner/Mazel, 2014.

Kerig, P. K. (2005). Revisiting the construct of boundary dissolution: A multidimensional perspective. *Journal of Emotional Abuse*, 1, 5–42. doi:10.4324/ 9781315821085–7

Kinet, M. (2008) *Ik weet niet hoe, ik weet niet waarom…we op elkaars systeem werken. In: Mark Kinet (Red.) Psychoanalyse en/van het Systeem. Bij jongeren en hun gezin.* Antwerpen/Apeldoorn: Garant.

Kinet, M. (2023). *The Spirit of the Drive in Neuropsychoanalysis.* London/New York: Routledge.

Kinet, M. (2024). *Psychoanalytic Principles in Psychiatric Practice. A Remedy by Truth*. London/New York: Routledge.

Klein, M. (1937). Love, guilt and reparation. In *Love, Guilt and Reparation and Other Works 1921–1945* (pp. 306–343). London: Virago, 1988.

Kohut, H. (1971). *The Analysis of the Self.* New York: International Universities Press.

Lacan, J. (1966). *Écrits.* Paris: Seuil.

Lyons-Ruth, K., Dutra, L., Schuder, M. and Boachi, I. (2006). From infant attachment disorganization to adult dissociation: relational adaptations or traumatic experience? *Psychiatric Clinics of North America*, 29, 63–86.

Macfie, J., Brumariu, L. E., and Lyons-Ruth, K. (2015). Parent–child role-confusion: A critical review of an emerging concept. *Developmental Review*, 36, 34–57. doi:10.1016/j.dr.2015.01.002

Madden, A. R., and Shaffer, A. (2016). Childhood parentification and adult relationship functioning. *Journal of Adult Development*, 23 (2), 90–102.

Masiran, N. A., Ibrahim, N., Nik Jaafar, N. R., and Siau, C. S. (2023). The positive and negative aspects of parentification: An integrated review. *Frontiers in Psychology*, 14, 1159739.

Minuchin, S. (1971). *Families and Family Therapy.* London/New York: Routledge, 1977.

Minuchin, S. (1981). *Family Therapy Techniques.* Cambridge, MA: Harvard University Press.

Napora, E. (2016). Parentification and grandparents' support from the perspective of grandchildren from families of various structures. *Acta Educationis Generalis*, 6 (1), 9–26.

Nehrig, N., Ho, S. S. M., and Wong, P. S. (2019). Understanding the self-object needs inventory: Its relationship to narcissism, attachment, and childhood maltreatment. *Psychoanalytic Psychology*, 36 (1), 53–63. doi:10.1037/pap0000182

Nuttall, A. K., Zhang, Q., Valentino, K., and Borkowski, J. G. (2019). Intergenerational risk of parentification and infantilization to externalizing moderated by child temperament. *Journal of Marriage and Family*, 81 (3), 648–661. doi:10.1111/jomf.12562

Onderwaater, A. (2009). *De onverbrekelijke band. Inleiding & ontwikkelingen in de contextuele therapie van Nagy.* Amsterdam: Pearson.

Oppenoorth, W. (1990). Parentificatie en projectieve identificatie. *Tijdschrift voor Psychotherapie*, 16, 25–35.

Oppenoorth, W. (1994). Parentificatie als ouderlijke projectieve identificatie. *Gezinstherapie*, 6 (1), 13–29.

Racker, H. (1968). *Transference and Countertransference.* London: Karnac, 1982.

Saha, A. (2016). Parentification: Boon or bane? *Journal of Psychological Research*, 11 (2), 289–301.

Sang, J., Cederbaum, J. A., and Hurlburt, M. S. (2014). Parentification, substance use, and sex among adolescent daughters from ethnic minority families. *Family Process*, 53 (2), 252–266. doi:10.1111/famp.12038

Schorr, S., and Goldner, L. (2023). 'Like stepping on glass': A theoretical model to understand the emotional experience of childhood parentification. *Family Relations*, 72(5), 3029–3048.

Shin, Y. J., and Hecht, M. L. (2013). Does parentification place Mexican-heritage youth at risk for substance use? Identifying the intervening nature of parent-child communication about alcohol. *Journal of Adolescence*, 36 (1), 149–159. doi:10.1016/j.adolescence.2012.10.010

Smith, J. A., Flowers, P., and Larkin, M. (2009). *Interpretative Phenomenological Analysis: Theory, Method and Research*. London: Sage.

Stein, G. L., Gonzalez, L. M., Cupito, A. M., Kiang, L., and Supple, A. J. (2015). The protective role of familism in the lives of Latino adolescents. *Journal of Family Issues*, 36(10), 1255–1273. doi:10.1177/0192513X13502480

Taillieu, T. L., Brownridge, D. A., Sareen, J., and Afifi, T. O. (2016). Childhood emotional maltreatment and mental disorders: Results from a nationally representative adult sample from the United States. *Child Abuse & Neglect*, 59, 1–12. doi:10.1016/j.chiabu.2016.07.005

Thastum, M., Johansen, M. B., Gubba, L., Olesen, L. B., and Romer, G. (2008). Coping, social relations, and communication: A qualitative exploratory study of children of parents with cancer. *Clinical Child Psychology and Psychiatry*, 13 (1), 123–138. doi:10.1177/1359104507086345

Thys, M. (2010). Tussen nijd en spijt. Parentificatie en reparatie. In M. Kinet (ed.) *Parentificatie. Als het kind te snel ouder wordt* (pp. 59–86). Antwerpen/Apeldoorn: Garant.

Tompkins, T. L. (2007). Parentification and maternal HIV infection: Beneficial role or pathological burden? *Journal of Child and Family Studies*, 16 (1), 108–118. doi:10.1007/s10826–10006–9072–9077

Valleau, M. P., Bergner, R. M., and Horton, C. B. (1995). Parentification and caretaker syndrome: An empirical investigation. *Family Therapy*, 22 (3), 157–164.

Van Buren, B. R., and Meehan, K. B. (2015). Child maltreatment and vulnerable narcissism: The roles of shame and disavowed need. *Journal of the American Psychoanalytic Association*, 63 (3), 555–561. doi:10.1177/0003065115593058

Van Loon, L. M. A., Van de Ven, M. O. M., Van Doesum, K. T. M., Hosman, C. M. H., and Witteman, C. L. M. (2017). Parentification, stress, and problem behavior of adolescents who have a parent with mental health problems. *Family Process*, 56 (1), 141–153. doi:10.1111/famp.12165

Van Mierlo, F., Michielsen, M., De Buysser, M. and Rooijakkers-Segers, G. (1998). Passend geven en nemen: hulpverlening aan volwassenen die als kind geparentificeerd werden. In M. Michielsen, W. van Mulligen and L. Hermkens (eds), *Leren over leven in loyaliteit. Over contextuele hulpverlening* (83–107). Leuven/Amersfoort: Acco.

Verhaeghe, P. (2009) *Het einde van de psychotherapie*. Amsterdam: Bezige Bij.

Williams, K., and Francis, S. E. (2010). Parentification and psychological adjustment: Locus of control as a moderating variable. *Contemporary Family Therapy*, 32(3), 231–237. doi:10.1007/s10591-010-9123-5

Winer, J. (1994). The parentified therapist. *Contemporary Psychoanalysis*, 30 (2), 297–314.

Winnicott, D. W. (1965). *The Maturational Processes and the Facilitating Environment: Studies in the Theory of Emotional Development*. London: Hogarth.

Chapter 6

Intermezzo II

Parentification: Clinical Vignette

A first clinical illustration shows the factor of parentification within a neurotic constellation with both pre-Oedipal and Oedipal components.

Isabel came for consultation because of fears and panic attacks that had been going on for many years. 'I don't dare to be alone.' For the past two years, obsessive thoughts have been added to this: 'I would hurt people. Especially people I love.' During the introductory conversation, she mentions that she 'expresses extremely positive feelings.' She always keeps herself cheerful and strong. She wants everything to go well everywhere. Negative feelings are—as it turns out—hardly ever expressed. Isabel has a senior administrative position. Her job frustrates her: she has many tasks and responsibilities, but is not allowed to make decisions. She feels hurt and wronged by her manager. She has already undergone psychotherapy with a female psychotherapist, but she is angry because she feels she did not receive enough attention and comfort from her.

Isabel is the eldest of three children. She has a 'very good relationship' with her parents. Her father is a labourer. 'I love him dearly.' As a little girl, he doted on her. She was also his pride and joy, whom he liked to show off to friends and colleagues. 'He took me out more than he took Mum.' She also recounts how nice it was when it was just the two of them when Mum was in the maternity ward before the birth of her younger brother. When there were arguments or tensions between her parents, Isabel always thought it was her fault. Her mother sometimes explicitly instructed her to appease her father and thus mediate in their conflicts. Her mother is initially described as somewhat bossy. But when Isabel was difficult or naughty, her mother did not get angry; she got sad. She cried. Isabel then felt very guilty. She also heard a lot about how her mother had gained a lot of weight as a result of her pregnancy, and that her stomach had become a 'battlefield' of stretch marks because of her.

Isabel says she was a cheerful and lively child. She tried hard to be an angel. In primary school, she always had to hear her mother's voice before she could go to class. After all, she had to check that her mother was still okay. During her adolescence, Isabel hardly rebelled at all. After six years of dating, she married a partner who was very much to her mother's liking, as

DOI: 10.4324/9781003645726-6

he was the ideal son-in-law. She sought security and stability in him. She herself was never really in love with him. The day after her wedding, she couldn't wait to return to her parental home. Until her wedding day, she had often slept in the same bed as her mother. Isabel had little interest in sex, and when it did happen, she didn't enjoy it much. She did have a few 'affairs,' however. That made her excited, and she was able to enjoy sex. Afterwards, though, she was left with a hangover.

During her clinical psychotherapeutic admission, she realised that she could no longer continue to be her mother's little angel. She came into contact with anger and other unwanted feelings that she had always anxiously and desperately hidden from her mother. In the ward, she rebelled and, feeling like she was at boarding school, got up to all sorts of mischief. Initially, impulsiveness reared its head and was strongly inhibited and/or suppressed, and she emerged as a flamboyant lady who, for example, dared to speak her mind in all kinds of small and large group meetings. Eventually, she even fell in love with a much younger, tough bad boy, with whom she began a 'forbidden' relationship (both by the ward rules and by her mother). She underwent a course of clinical psychotherapy lasting about a year and a half. She left in good spirits and immediately (and continuously since then) resumed her work. Since then, she has been undergoing weekly psychoanalytic therapy.

Over time, it has become abundantly clear that she struggles with a great deal of anger and even murderous impulses, which she keeps (over)covered under a thick cloak of love. The return of what was repressed leads to obsessive symptoms such as aggressive or sadistic compulsive thoughts towards 'innocents.' She has particular difficulty with delicate, sensitive individuals. She acts overly empathetic and caring towards them precisely because they get on her nerves (just like her mother). 'Sometimes I could pin them to the wall.' On the other hand, in her professional life or in traffic, for example, she is a very combative and tough woman who sometimes looks for '*trouble*' to vent her pent-up aggression, even towards complete strangers. Her compulsions are not only aggressive but also sexual in nature. For example, she compulsively checks whether she has become involuntarily wet vaginally.

Initially, she saw herself as a victim of her mother's emotional blackmail. She felt defenceless against her tears, which she considered a powerful and effective weapon. From her stories, her mother emerges as an egocentric woman with low self-esteem. Her younger brothers never let themselves be 'caught' by their mother's (in their eyes melodramatic) fuss (and still don't to this day). They make short work of it and quickly go their own way. Isabel, on the other hand, feels that from an early age she has been 'called upon' to cheer her up and be her ray of sunshine. She plays an important role in her mother's self-esteem and must constantly affirm her as a fantastic mother. After school, until after puberty, a hot chocolate would await her, which she was supposed to drink cosily with her mother, while she would rather have been hanging out with her friends (with or without mopeds) at the school gate. While she is there for her mother, or *is supposed* to be, she feels misunderstood and/or abandoned by her mother in moments of emotional distress. As if it is always only *her* feelings that matter most.

In addition to these pre-Oedipal components, over the years, Isabel also becomes more aware of rival feelings towards her mother. She secretly triumphed over her mother and enjoyed being able to wrap her father (but also other father figures) around her little finger. There are unconscious feelings of guilt and a need for punishment for the damage she caused her mother. She gradually comes to realise that she was very seductive, but in a subtle, camouflaged way. She often referred to a white, sleeveless (men's) undershirt that made her look boyish but showed off her two assets to the male population.

In therapy, she is very sensitive to empathic deficits. This may be linked to how she always experienced her mother. Due to repeated violence, she was able to break away from her *bad boy* shortly after her admission. She was assisted in this by her current partner. He too had/has a 'smell' (he is a cannabis-smoking, unemployed man who spends his days doing nothing at home, but who, viewed positively, functions as a househusband by the fireside). On the other hand, he is dependent on her and 'carries me on his hands' (an expression she also used with her father). Isabel is, in his eyes, above all other women and therefore has no competition to fear. The Oedipal prohibition, the punishment, and the need for emotional care and narcissistic gratification find their apparent satisfaction in this symptomatic choice of partner for a while. For Isabel, these cards were on the table, but for years, it was her 'conscious' choice to play this game. Meanwhile, her partner's cannabis addiction steadily escalated. He now embodied the fragile and sensitive mother who, like a puppy in distress (which she frequently brought into the house), needed to be cared for. Then he stood for the father who made her feel loved, cherished, and adored, and who waited for her in the evening with candles and tea lights.

For years, Isabel appeared indestructibly cheerful in our conversations. She would stay away for longer periods of time, and afterwards it always turned out that incidents of aggression had occurred because of her partner, in which he threatened murder and suicide, and she sometimes had to flee to the neighbours. It was as if (as with her mother) she only wanted to show me her best side and solve all her problems herself and alone. Only little by little did it become clear how much she was being terrorised by his emotional problems. She started working full-time and, because of her partner's social anxiety, had to do all the shopping and take care of all the practical matters. She had chronic money problems because he (literally) blew so much money on drugs, and she sometimes had to put herself in dangerous situations to find his 'stuff' in environments that were not always kosher. Meanwhile, she hid the extent of the problems from the outside world (and not least from her parents). She compared herself to a fairy who could perform magic or to

Mega Mindy, a Wonder Woman in a pink costume who was all over some children's TV channels at the time. She was especially afraid of being accused of it being all her own fault. Why did she let it get this far? Why didn't she leave her partner? She would have been better off staying with her husband instead of leaving him for 'bad' men. After yet another threat, which required the intervention of a colleague (who happened to be visiting) and the police, her partner was finally admitted to the hospital. He underwent a long period of withdrawal treatment and has since returned to work for the first time since he got together with Isabel. He remains 'clean' and his attitude and behaviour towards Isabel are exemplary. He seems to realise (and also wants to make amends for) what he has done to her all this time.

Meanwhile, her parents moved into a flat due to reduced mobility, and her father died shortly afterwards. Isabel described her mother during the period of illness that preceded this in similar terms to before: egocentric and uninvolved. She told a whole story about a garden gnome she had once gone to buy with her father. For her, it embodied their shared poetic-romantic disposition and the special relationship that existed between father and daughter. Her mother had never understood these kinds of things very well. Because she had unceremoniously removed the garden gnome from the balcony of their terrace and put it out with the rubbish, she was portrayed as a heartless, but also superficial creature, completely oblivious to the finer expressions of emotional life.

It is remarkable how her view of her parents has changed since then. In recent years, her mother has become a kind of *Lustige Witwe* (merry widow). Despite her advanced age, she is more coquettish and feminine than ever. She also goes out a lot: she visits museums, theatre performances, and even exotic cities and regions. Isabel has had many conversations with her mother and has had to drastically adjust her image of her parents as a result. It turns out that her parents courted for a long time and still had a very passionate relationship. They waited a long time to have children because they wanted to enjoy each other's company for long enough. Her mother had to stay at home to look after the children, under pressure from her father. Her father worked a lot and was often away from home, leaving all the parenting to his wife. Only he did the fun and enjoyable things with and for the children. He suffered from the loss of exclusive attention and could isolate himself and sulk in a childish manner. Isabel felt called upon (and, over time, also by her mother) to mediate, break the ice, and help her father come around. More and more, Isabel came to the conclusion that she apparently felt guilty simply because she *was* there; she felt that her birth had made her parents unhappy in their own way, and that it was her mission to make up for this unconscious crime. She did this by wanting to be her father's princess and her mother's angel. On closer inspection, she had been engaged in a kind of *Mission Impossible* her entire life. The price she paid for this was that all negative/inappropriate feelings had to be kept out of contact and only expressed in obsessive thoughts with a high (literally and figuratively) "Fuck!" content. In therapy, she was able to behave in a very regressive manner. She made a lot of appeals (even between sessions) and at times acted very helpless and dependent. Mega Mindy turned into Mini Mindy, and various issues that had been rejected by her mother could now be mentalised and discussed.

Chapter 7

Twist in My Sobriety

Parentification and Alcohol

Introduction

Alcohol abuse has far-reaching consequences, not only for the drinker but also for those around them. Research shows that partners, children, and wider social circles suffer from the physical, psychological and social effects of problematic drinking.[1] Adult Children of Alcoholics (ACA) is the term used to describe adults who grew up in a family with alcohol problems. They often exhibit recurring patterns in relationships, self-image, and dependency, which influence their psychological development.[2] Children who grow up in families where alcohol abuse plays a dominant role are indeed often marked for life by the psychological consequences. These adults form a group that is recognisable in epidemiological studies by their increased vulnerability to psychiatric disorders, relational instability, reduced school performance, behavioural problems, and self-destructive tendencies.[3] From a psychoanalytical perspective, this is understood in terms of disturbed attachment, internalisation of destructive object relations, and repetition compulsion. Recent large-scale cohort studies confirm the increased risks of mood and anxiety disorders, substance abuse, and premature mortality.[4] However, figures alone do not provide insight into the problem's inner logic. Here, psychoanalysis opens a deeper window: it examines how, for example, early childhood relational trauma, identification with the parent's symptom, or inadequate containment disrupt the psychological reality of ACA. This chapter brings together epidemiological and empirical findings with insights from Freud, Ferenczi, Klein, Winnicott, Bion, and Lacan to arrive at an integrated understanding of typical ACA problems.

Epidemic

In a sense, alcohol is epidemic. According to the World Health Organisation, approximately 10% of the population in Europe and the US has an alcohol problem.[5] On the other hand, it is estimated that more than 50% of children from families with substance abuse or dependence are parentified.[6] In the under-15 age group, approximately one in ten children live in a family where

DOI: 10.4324/9781003645726-7

one or both parents have an alcohol problem. Estimates range from 12% to 27% at home and abroad.[7] In Ireland, for example, around 12% of the population is said to be parentified as a result of alcohol. A study into the harmful effects of alcohol on others shows that three in five respondents had a heavy drinker in their lives, and one in ten testified that children were victims of this in the form of physical and verbal abuse, being left in unsafe situations and/or exposure to serious forms of aggression.[8] Of the children receiving mental health treatment in Sweden, 87% have a parent with an addiction and/or psychiatric problem. This is probably representative of all Western European countries.[9]

When families with substance abuse problems are followed over three generations, it appears that in all these families at least one of the children took on a parental role, thereby compensating for the absent or inadequate parent (usually the father). They also found that such children often had parenting difficulties with their own children and tended to abuse substances when they encountered stressful life situations in adulthood. These children had an excessive sense of responsibility that extended into their adult lives.[10] When one of the parents is addicted to alcohol, there is indeed a much greater chance of parentification than in cases of alcohol abuse.[11] Children with a drinking mother reported more parentification than children with a drinking father. There also appear to be more gender-specific differences in parentification. Daughters who mainly suspect their mother of problem drinking feel more parentified.[12] When the father has an alcohol problem, daughters seem to have more difficulty with their identity development and with sustained commitment to their careers or relationships.[13] They are therefore less focused on personal happiness and success.[14]

Comparative research consistently shows that both instrumental and emotional parentification are more common in alcoholic families than in non-alcoholic families.[15] There also appears to be a clear correlation between alcoholism or other substance abuse by parents and the experience of parentification by children and young people.[16] Moreover, there is a proportional relationship between the two: the more alcohol, the more parentification.[17] Various studies have shown that families of alcoholics are more disorganised and conflictual, and also have reduced cohesion. There is also an increased risk of poverty, divorce, unemployment and chaos.[18] In approximately 20% of cases of child abuse, alcohol abuse is also involved.[19] Alcohol plays a role in 50 to 70% of families where incest and child sexual abuse occur.[20]

Empirical

The unpredictability within the family that accompanies alcoholism may be the main pathogenic factor. Inconsistent parenting, a lack of fixed family rituals, and socio-economic instability mean that children often feel lonely and emotionally overwhelmed. By caring for the alcohol-dependent parent, they gain a false sense of control and can ward off feelings of fear and helplessness.[21] Of course, secure attachment is also hampered by parental substance abuse. In the ambivalent-insecure type, contradictory or unpredictable parenting plays a major role, while in disorganised attachment, emotional co-regulation is lacking. Everyone today probably agrees that the latter causes a complex and serious disruption of all fundamental biopsychosocial competencies. The unpredictable and frightening behaviour associated with parental substance abuse can cause symptoms similar to those of post-traumatic stress disorder. In young children, for example, it can lead to bedwetting, sleep disorders, and rocking (themselves).[22] The effect on later school performance is debatable. On the one hand, these children may be more prone to fighting, bullying, or other signs of aggression, but on the other hand, school can also be a safe haven for them. After all, their school performance can also benefit or restore their self-image. Neglect or a lack of parental supervision can be very damaging to a child's self-esteem. All these negative consequences can remain under the radar for a long time. Not least because of the taboo and atmosphere of secrecy that surrounds alcohol problems, even though they are the 'organising principle' par excellence of the household.[23]

Against their will, children are both witnesses and victims of moments or episodes of conflict, separation, attacks, or domestic violence. What often occurs with alcoholic parent(s) is inconsistent parenting, unpredictable rules and boundaries, a chaotic or tense atmosphere, poor communication, broken promises, and loneliness or isolation related to the need or obligation to keep the problem secret/hidden from the outside world in order to avoid embarrassment or shame. The lack of predictability causes mixed feelings in the child and disrupts their sense of security, leading to long-term stress and reduced resistance or resilience.[24]

Research shows that children as young as eighteen months suffer from their parents' alcohol problems. They have higher levels of aggression, and these levels do not decrease with age, unlike those in a non-alcoholic control group. They have less self-regulation. This is evident from preschool age in their interactions with their environment, and also reduces their cognitive abilities.[25] As a result, they are more likely to have lower school performance and exhibit psychopathology, diagnosable psychiatric disorders, learning difficulties, eating disorders, or perfectionism. Emotionally, they are somewhat distrustful and have an excessive need for control and responsibility. They have a deep-rooted belief that they must care for others at all costs.[26] They display a resilience that prevents them from engaging in self-destructive behaviour, but the question is whether not being able to let loose or 'go wild' at all is a sign of 'healthy' behaviour…

The Alcoholic Personality

In order to properly understand the impact of an alcoholic parent on a child, I will first take a closer look at the alcoholic personality.[27] Alcoholism is one of the most complex and widespread forms of addiction. Traditional medical and behavioural models often describe it in terms of dependence, habit formation, or neurobiological vulnerability.[28] While most people can use chemical products in moderation, for some, substance use becomes excessive and/or transgressive. They are greedy and immoderate in their relationship with the product and can no longer stop. They are aware of the harmful and potentially lethal consequences of their use, but the substance has become a necessity for them, to which they are driven with longing.

For some, the substance has become a narcotic. The intoxication mainly brings oblivion and, as such, becomes the only and immediate solution to all negative feelings and problems. Intoxication is indeed a way of compensating for a lack of mentalising ability or of short-circuiting mentalisation. Unbearable contents are evacuated rather than thought about, let alone verbalised. In psychopathology that corresponds more to the deficit model than to the conflict model, in what Peter Fonagy calls mental process disorders[29] and what Paul Verhaeghe considers to be actual pathology,[30] substance use is the ideal way to free oneself from all kinds of unspeakable tensions or stimuli. For example, in the case of trauma, alcoholic brainwashing may be the only way out of a shocking, degrading, and/or desubjectivising story. It is a spectacular illustration of the indispensable place that intoxicants can occupy in the inner workings of the mind. They serve to numb all kinds of psychological pain instead of '*suffering the process of thinking*.'[31]

For others, the substance is more of a stimulant that captivates them and whose taste never leaves them. In an allusion to snorting cocaine, intoxication can be a direct line drawn to the Thing. The result is a mythical enjoyment, the nostalgic rediscovery of total satisfaction. Sándor Rado, one of the psychoanalytic pioneers in the analysis of substance use, spoke of the pharmacogenic orgasm. It is an orgasm that is within reach as a *jouissance à volonté* through the intake of a product. He compares it to the essentially oral orgasm of the baby at the mother's breast.[32] In that sense, the nipple is our first heroin, notre première héroïne. And these first oral experiences of satisfaction serve as a model for our later longing for a mythical and symbiotic jouissance, as conceived by the Lacanians. With alcohol as a narcotic or stimulant, the person ventures beyond good and evil, beyond healthy and unhealthy behaviour, in search of destructive enjoyment. He has become dependent on a single solution or a slave to a single impossible, forbidden, and excessive enjoyment.

Freudian

In Freud's writings, references to substance use are very sporadic. In a letter to Fliess dated 22 December 1897, he establishes a link between alcohol intoxication and masturbation.[33] In this letter, he refers to the latter as a primal urge for which alcohol intoxication serves as a substitute. In his essay on jokes, he states that alcohol removes inhibitions, improves mood, and reduces self-criticism.[34] In his three treatises published that same year, he considers substance use to be an oral fixation or perversion.[35] In his analysis of the connection between mourning and melancholy, he ultimately compares intoxication to mania and manic defence.[36] Here and there in his work, we also find the view that frustration of the demand for love leads to regression—for example, in the form of comfort sought in satisfying the need. The person concerned begins to eat, drink, or sleep excessively.

According to epidemiological data, at least one personality disorder can be diagnosed in 60% of the psychiatric population with substance abuse or dependence problems.[37] Personality disorders apparently form a fertile breeding ground in which later substance abuse can germinate.

Based on all the psychoanalytical literature and from a so-called classical Freudian perspective, Fenichel characterised the so-called pre-morbid addictive personality as follows in the middle of the last century.[38] These are patients who easily give up their object love because they have never been good at developing relationships with others. They are fixated on passive-receptive instinctual goals. Substance abusers also have little or no interest in the particularities or personality of their partner. Their capacity for giving is limited and they have little regard for reality. Erotic pleasure is often less important to them than ways to increase their self-esteem or maintain their sense of self. Everyone will undoubtedly recognise Heinz Kohut's theories in this description, in which the patient uses the other person as a self-object to maintain a positive and cohesive narcissistic balance.[39]

(Post-)Kleinian

In a more Kleinian line of thinking, Edward Glover considers substance use as a defence against depressive anxieties or psychotic fragmentation.[40] He emphasises the importance of a pre-genital sadistic fixation in this pathology. The dependency product is used to kill, punish, or neutralise the poorly internalised object, or to ward off the threat posed by a poorly projected object. For him, substance use is essentially a form of self-treatment in the absence of an adequate defence against certain affects. This is a narcissistic disorder that is further characterised by pathology of the superego, by an inadequate capacity for symbolisation and by dependence on archaic (i.e. early childhood) objects. For most Kleinians, the product symbolises an ideal, magical, and omnipotent object that provides immediate pleasure while apparently independent of external reality. The intoxication is characterised by narcissistic regression and an artificial, pharmacogenic mania in which phenomena such as idealisation, identification with the ideal object, and omnipotent control of this object play a central role.

Herbert Rosenfeld believes that alcoholics have only a weak ego that cannot tolerate pain, frustration, or depression.[41] All fears and frustrations are denied through a manic defence mechanism. The bad and aggressive parts of the self are split off, and the pharmacotoxic effect reinforces mechanisms of omnipotent control, denial, and splitting. The addiction serves to avoid or break through an affective dependence on significant others. It is an escape from the depressive position with the recognition of dependence and the fear of loss and abandonment that accompanies it. Anyone who visits an alcohol withdrawal unit is struck by the jolly pub-without-beer atmosphere, where patients continue to chat jovially and cheerfully even though they are up to their ears in shit. The persistent, sometimes even ridiculous tendency to lie and deny, as well as the almost delusional exteriorisation in which all evil is situated outside themselves, is also exemplary of Kleinian schizoid-paranoid functioning.

According to Wilfred Bion's theory, thinking can only develop to the extent that the child's perceptions are digested and translated by the Big Other.[42] This happens through processes of projective identification, whereby the child or patient makes the Other feel something unbearable and calls on that Other as a kind of translation machine. The maternal psyche, with its containment and reverie, provides the necessary transformation in the child's mentalising capacity. Mutatis mutandis, we can describe intoxication in Bionian terms as a transformation into hallucinosis that attacks thinking, destroys bonds and connections, and creates the illusion of a world of one's own in false omniscience (-L[ove], -K[knowledge], -H[ate]).[43]

In line with Winnicott, Joyce McDougall considers addiction to be a neo-need. This is a pathology of the transitional object.[44] As is well known, this transitional object is a blanket, rug, toy, or teddy bear that takes on a special, vitally important meaning for the child and helps bridge the absence of the mother. In a sense, the transitional object can be regarded as a structuring object of addiction. It is a subjective object created by the child with the mother's cooperation. It allows the child to detach from the mother without denying her absence. The transitional object symbolises the mother and allows the child to internalise her as a protective object. However, if the first major Other fails in its containing and transformative function, the child seeks refuge in a transitional object that allows it to deny the mother's absence. This transitional object is temporary and transient. It offers no real support because it must always be found; it is always out there. This transitional object can lead to disinvestment in the long, difficult and painful process of holding on and letting go, of being together and of separation. It creates a kind of shunt, a short circuit.[45] There is no linguistic, symbolic or psychological elaboration. On the contrary, the person concerned becomes more and more absorbed in or submerged by a progressively more inhuman, stereotypical, sterile and desolate toxicomaniac behaviour, as is poignantly shown, for example, in the feature film *Requiem for a Dream.*[46]

What happens here is therefore the opposite of mourning with its endless letting go of the object. And this is extremely harmful to development because people must accept loss in order to find themselves and discover the object in its radical otherness.[47] In the ideology of addiction, postponement and desire are crushed under the need for immediate satisfaction of a need. 'I want it all and I want it now!' The lack of and craving for the product masks a deeper lack of being or a lack of having. There is also a danger of forgetting that substance use essentially refers to a transgression of the law (of the incest taboo and the pleasure principle).[48]

French Psychoanalysis

Lacanians will emphasise, in particular, that the father has not been able to instil investment in the realm of scarcity and desire. This is nevertheless necessary in order to open up a space between mother and child and between inner and outer reality. For many addicts, the father is absent or conflict-averse. He is too egalitarian or too authoritarian, he is inconsistent or transgressive. It is not uncommon for him to be a substance user himself. Of all the post-Freudians, Lacan is the only one who takes the Oedipus complex and castration out of the closet and gives them a new linguistic twist. He presents the father, the law, and language as structuring elements and, in addition to separation and individuation, he puts forward sexuation as a stumbling block.

The user of resources avoids confrontation with the sexual Other and takes the shortest route to a form of enjoyment that lies beyond language and is separate from, and precedes, gender difference.[49] From a Lacanian perspective, there are indeed two forms of enjoyment. The first form is safe, limited and belongs to the phallic-Oedipal order. These are the small things (*'les bien'*) in life. We are allowed to enjoy them, and we can enjoy them. In addition, there is a desire for total and unlimited enjoyment of an unnameable and unimaginable Thing. This Thing is a good ('le Bien') that is at the same time a 'mal,' as in Baudelaire's 'Les fleurs du Mal.' It is a forbidden and impossible Thing that is destructive to desire and subjectivity. Drug addiction is the search for excessive enjoyment that necessarily leads to (premature) death.[50]

A well-known Jenny Holzer slogan reads: 'Protect me from what I want.'[51] It is an appeal to the second great Other, namely the father who, through his law, intervenes not repressively but protectively, erecting a dam against a bottomless and all-consuming archaic enjoyment. After all, the addict avoids the detour via the Other and the mediating influence of language. He abandons limited enjoyment and radically opts for immediate, yet forbidden, access to *jouissance*. Lacanians do not speak of addiction but of a-diction.[52] The addict cultivates an illusory enjoyment that eludes castration (as understood by Lacan). In doing so, however, the addict inevitably enters the realm of death and the death drive.

According to French psychoanalyst Jean Bergeret, there is no separate drug addict personality structure.[53] However, he does believe that many drug addicts share a number of common traits, such as a *lack* of mental processing, a *poverty* of the imaginary and a tendency to *act out*. His compatriot Michèle

Monjauze, on the other hand, has developed an original and influential approach: she sees alcoholism as a specific psychopathological organisation, distinct from both neurosis and psychosis.[54] For Monjauze, alcoholism is more than a behavioural problem or an impulse control disorder. It is a structural organisation of the psychic apparatus characterised by a split within the self. On the one hand, there is an adaptive part that functions within the social and linguistic order: the patient can work, talk, reason, and apparently integrate. On the other hand, there is an 'alcoholic part' that functions regressively, escapes symbolic mediation, and operates on a preverbal, sensory, and affective level.[55] According to Monjauze, alcohol acts as a psychological prosthesis that must dampen unbearable affects: fears of emptiness, loss of object relations, or a catastrophic collapse of the self.[56] Drinking is, therefore, less a conscious choice than a necessity to protect the regressive part from disintegration. This also explains the stubbornness and resistance to change.

Monjauze locates the roots of alcoholism in early experiences of deprivation in the parent-child relationship. Insufficient mirroring, inadequate holding, or inconsistent affective contact can lead to a deficit in the development of a stable sense of self. Alcohol later appears as a substitute for the missing internal object that should guarantee security and coherence.[57] Monjauze does not place alcoholism in the realm of repression, but rather in that of falsification and splitting. Whereas Freud emphasised the conflict between instinct and prohibition, Monjauze emphasises the fundamental vulnerability of the self that precedes conflict. According to her, alcohol can temporarily alleviate this rupture: it provides an artificial illusion of security and integration. Drinking thus becomes a 'liquid holding environment' that compensates for the failing psychological framework. Countertransference is also important. Monjauze warns that alcoholics often evoke intense feelings of powerlessness, irritation, or fascination in those around them or their therapist.[58] This is in line with the observations of my Lacanian compatriots Stijn Vanheule and Paul Verhaeghe, who link alcoholism to narcissistic structures in which the therapist can easily become entangled.[59]

In the Shadow of the Bottle

I will now focus more closely on the specific experiences of those who grow up in the shadow of alcoholism. These experiences stem from a number of specific characteristics of the alcoholic personality described above. The clinical addictive personality presents itself as an infantile organisation, determined by a number of primitive modes of functioning.[60] These manifest as the following behavioural characteristics: poor affect control, which manifests itself on the one hand through increased impulsivity (aggressiveness, low frustration tolerance, discontinuous behaviour patterns, etc.) and on the other hand through increased compulsivity (immediate and total need satisfaction, need for power, etc.); and mental and cognitive rigidity, which manifests itself on the one hand through a lack of cognitive generalisation and creativity, and on the other hand through a weak mentalisation ability, especially at the second level. Addicts have little mental space: mental representation, understanding, and symbolisation are rather limited. Emotional flattening and egocentrism are evident in limited empathy and superficial sentimentality. The experience of a 'deficit' can often be traced back to the experience of a lack of pleasure and intoxication. Primitive defence mechanisms, mainly denial, splitting, projection, and reversal: these defence systems 'protect' the addict from confronting his dysfunction and his anxiety. Increased frequency of personality disorders: in a number of patients, we see the addictive behaviour coexisting with a pre-existing personality disorder through one of the following patterns: the schizoid-paranoid mode (aggression, jealousy, isolation), the dependent-depressive mode (boundlessness, dependence), the narcissistic-isolated mode (need for power and competition, theatricality) and the obsessive-compulsive mode (control, perfectionism, and excessive criticality). Parallel to the healthy ego, the addict develops a toxic ego, giving the personality a dual structure, as it were. When the addiction becomes chronic, the split often becomes more permanent. It should be noted that the toxic ego remains active even during the sober phase. It often uses denial, splitting, projection, and reversal as primitive defence mechanisms that protect against confronting one's own dysfunction. Cognitive changes are noticeable through a decline or change in consciousness. Judgement weakens so that disparate elements can be taken into account less. Genuine consultation or dialogue becomes difficult. On an affective level, a combination of apathy and emotional instability occurs. When the parent is under the influence, unprocessed events often surface that are never discussed when sober. Alcohol, due to its disinhibiting effect, reduces both impulse control and frustration tolerance, resulting in more frequent aggressive outbursts and violence. Increasing conflicts within the relationship, along with the additional worries of the non-drinking partner, contribute to blurred boundaries. Due to the deteriorating course of substance abuse, the parents are left with a 'deficit' and the child feels compelled to fill the growing deficit in parallel. Taking on this parental role is often the only form of closeness that the child can still experience with their parent. The asymmetrical relationship between parent and child, as an existential given, is gradually ignored or even reversed. An addicted parent or their partner can be very intrusive and/or take over the child's psychological space. The child identifies with this parental role, leading them to miss out on connections, experiences, and skill development in their personal life. If the drinking continues for a longer period of time, the family will try to control and shield the problem.

The child tries to control the use by, for example, counting the number of drinks consumed or putting marks on bottles. Unfortunately, caring for the addicted parent rarely causes the parent to stop using. Often, the parent promises to stop but fails to do so, or only manages to do so for a limited period. The child often feels guilty and incompetent because they cannot achieve what they so desperately want. This usually leads to a negative self-image and feelings of inferiority, which cause even more endless worry. Exhaustion and symptoms of depression pile up. The child shows great empathy, but also a lack of awareness of their own needs and desires. They continue to feel disappointed in the other person, who never gives back in kind, causing a sense of injustice to build silently. The child who must remain a child remains dependent out of loyalty to the parent's need for care. The 'sick child' is a variant of this form of parentification. The perfect child will focus on meeting all of the parents' expectations. High-level functioning can be seen as a 'means' of making them feel good about themselves. In this way, an early form of workaholism can develop. Because competition and the pursuit of a career are considered important in our society, this form of 'addiction' often goes unnoticed. Important protective factors in all this are the support of the non-drinking parent, regular and stable family rituals, a good relationship with siblings, and/or support from the community to which the family belongs.[61]

ACA Psychodynamic

Now that the prevalence, relevance, and perception of parentification in ACA have been sufficiently explained, I will delve into the underlying psychodynamics. Chronic unpredictability, emotional neglect, and, more generally, failed parenting go hand in hand with implicit rules of secrecy, denial, and impasse, leading to what Salvador Minuchin called enmeshment and boundary confusion. From a psychoanalytical perspective, the child's ego becomes prematurely organised around defence mechanisms such as reaction formation, repression, and identification with the aggressor.[62] The child loses touch with its own emotions and motivations because it is primarily attuned to the parents' affective state, which is scanned and monitored in a permanent state of hypervigilance. The role reversal disrupts the development of the ego and self, distorts or damages the construction of object relations and creates patterns of problematic relationship formation. Parentification becomes internalised and becomes an integral part of the person concerned's mindset. It places an emotional yoke on that person.[63] It creates a kind of default mode that unfolds unconsciously/automatically throughout adulthood. It is a programming error that becomes installed and, like any involuntary symptom, it is a place of suffering and (often strange) enjoyment. It causes gain and loss. It was once a creative invention/solution, but over time, its automation has become more disadvantageous than advantageous.

The long-term effects of the processes described are complex and manifold. Classically, a pathological superego develops: exaggerated feelings of guilt and responsibility are the echoes of a strict parent who constantly scolds the child so that it disregards or sacrifices its own interests for the benefit of this increasingly demanding Big Other. The sense of self is disturbed by premature role reversal and blurred boundaries. The child remains under the spell of idealised or haunting inner objects, with all the negative consequences this entails for intimacy, dependence, and attachment in their adult relationships. Last but not least, the compulsion to repeat takes its toll. Old interactions and dynamics in which self-loss and co-dependence play a major role come back to life on stage.[64]

Meta-analyses show a limited but consistent correlation between parental substance use and insecure attachment.[65] According to attachment theory, the quality of the early parent-child relationship forms a blueprint for adulthood. As mentioned above, the three forms of insecure attachment (avoidant, ambivalent, or disorganised) are common in ACA.[66] This is related to the inconsistencies described, such as aggression. All this complicates later romantic relationships, given the fear of intimacy, mistrust, and low self-esteem that results from it.[67] As parents, ACA (especially females) are often overprotective, very stressed about raising their children and doubt their own abilities.[68] Object relations theorists such as Fairbairn, Klein and Winnicott emphasise how internal images of the first others leave their mark on the self and further relationships.[69] In order to maintain a 'good' image of the parent (s), the child takes the blame upon itself.[70] This leads to feelings of guilt and shame, as well as low self-esteem and feelings of inferiority. The child works hard to make up for and keep (the parent) happy. Melanie Klein's concept of the depressive position is also relevant here: ACA carry guilt and fear the parental object for having damaged it with their own aggression.[71] The unconscious guilt that results from this makes them feel compelled as adults to repair the damage and makes them vulnerable to depressive disorders.

A sufficiently long period of dependence is necessary for optimal development, but ACA develop excessive self-reliance and deny normal and healthy needs for support, resulting in isolation. Others are clingy and seek constant closeness, or they react with hostility to any sense of dependence. An intoxicated parent is emotionally absent. The child lacks a mirror and a sounding board. At such times, Winnicott's good-enough mother is compromised, and the child experiences not attunement but abandonment. It is not a containing presence that is stored but a broken and inconsistent 'object,' resulting not in sand as a foundation but rather quicksand. Dependency is a normal developmental phenomenon, but in ACA, it is disrupted in various ways.

ACA show a higher risk of developing substance dependence themselves.[72] This is usually associated with hereditary factors, but, from a psychoanalytical perspective, identification processes can also be held responsible. Even before Freud, identification was considered the first form of emotional bond.[73] The child becomes (like) the parent in order to forge the bond. In the case of alcoholism, the child may repeat this symptom of the parent out of a sense of loyalty. Ferenczi's concept of the confusion of languages between adults and children is also relevant here.[74] The child is drawn into and overwhelmed by adult psychodynamics. The ACA, who drink, can be understood as proof of loyalty and a desperate attempt to counter the incomprehensible emotional absence of the parent. With the bottle within reach, everything remains 'under control.' The best and most reliable friends become, so to speak, Jack Daniel's or Johnnie Walker is a variation on Jacques Lacan's *le partenaire-symptôme.*[75] The parental drink takes the place of the Thing around which desire and enjoyment gravitate. The child orients itself via this Thing, and the bottle becomes, as it were, a surrogate partner. It refers to the way in which the other (the partner in love or the analytical partner) functions as the bearer or embodiment of the subject's symptom, thereby making its existence bearable. After all, in a sense, it guarantees the continuity of one's own psychic organisation: by loving what hurts, one's subjective structure remains intact. The analytical work consists not so much in correcting this 'flawed' love object, but in understanding it and reworking the relationship to it. Epidemiological research shows that ACA are more likely than the broader young adult population to not participate in education, training, and employment. They apparently have more difficulty fitting into the social order. From a Lacanian perspective, this may be related to the fact that the paternal function is insufficiently established. As a result of emotional absence or unpredictability, the alcoholic parent does not or insufficiently represents the Name and the No of the father. The symbolic law that should help the child enter the domains of language, culture, and desire is lacking. As a result, the child remains at the mercy of whims and caprices. In the absence of the mediating and regulating role of the symbolic, it remains prey to chaos or the inertia and impasses of a deadly repetition.

In the ACA, we also find more frequent self-harming behaviour and premature mortality. From a psychoanalytical point of view, the work of the death drive, introduced by Freud in the context of a compulsion to repeat and a tendency towards entropy or decomposition with a return to the 'dead' inorganic state, may play a role here. In ACA, self-destruction can function as an unconscious attempt to reunite with the parent: an act of fidelity and loyalty to the lost or damaged object. The Bionian nameless dread associated with a lack of containment is evacuated in a self-destructive enactment in which what is beyond comprehension is acted out.[76] Mutatis mutandis, mentalising and symbolising developmental support are necessary here to break these destructive patterns.

Finally, an important factor in the ACA is the shame and stigma of addiction that children of alcoholic parents secretly carry with them.[77] Valuable inspiration is provided here by the concept of the psychological crypt: that which cannot or must not be spoken of (the parent's alcohol problem, intrafamilial violence) is sealed and passed on between the lines to the next generation.[78] They must bear this unspeakable secret, while it silently underlies symptoms and patterns that, like hardware, escape interpretation.

Psychotherapy

The advantage of psychodynamic and psychogenetic diagnostics is that they provide inherent starting points for treatment. Under the motto 'prevention is better than cure,' contemporary addiction care often pays appropriate attention to psychoeducation from the outset. For alcoholic parents, their partners, and children, it provides an overview so that they can see the forest for the trees that previously escaped their attention. In a manner and with means appropriate to their age and level, the children are heard and recognised (often for the first time) for the precarious position they find themselves in. This in itself has therapeutic value. Family-oriented interventions are effective. Interventions that involve not only the child but the whole family (parents, children, communication) often have even stronger outcomes.[79] Communication about mental health problems is both crucial and complex. Parents struggle with what, when, and how to tell their children about their mental illness. They experience shame, guilt, and uncertainty, and want to protect their children.[80] Clinical teams rarely ask what children already know or provide guidance on how to communicate, even though parents are usually open to this. Of the five key protective factors identified to help strengthen resilience, information and social support are at the top of the list.[81]

This psychoeducation can be an eye-opener for both the alcoholic parent(s) and their child(ren). It creates an awareness of the problem, which can naturally lead to a request for psychotherapeutic help. In children and young people, psychotherapy always requires some integration between a systemic and a psychoanalytical perspective, both to understand the problem and to treat it. This will be discussed in more detail in the next chapter.

With ACA, a number of therapeutic guidelines logically read as follows. Firstly, a kind of mourning process is needed for the loss of a carefree childhood that was insufficient (or sometimes even non-existent). As children, we are 'naturally' entitled to this, and when we were unable to experience it, we feel that we have been wronged and that sooner or later this must be acknowledged, if not remedied. Secondly, the object relations that populate our inner world must be reconstructed, i.e., the main characters that determine our inner theatre. In particular, there must be more distinction between me and you, the self and the other. Thirdly, excessive feelings of guilt and responsibility must be tempered. More technically speaking, the parentified person must try to free themselves from a punitive superego, mainly through interpretations and the resulting increased insight into the origin and existence of these torments. Fourthly, help must be given to build a cohesive self in which manifestations of the true self are recognised and affirmed, so that authentic desires and feelings are given the space they need to escape the yoke of a false self. All this can only take place within the holding and facilitating environment of the psychotherapeutic relationship(s), where sufficient safety is consistently provided to be able/dare to expose oneself and to recover sufficiently. The corrective emotional experience advocated and embodied in this way can be internalised, and repetition, repetition, repetition and working through, working through, working through are necessary to get old patterns out and new ones into our 'system.'

Certainly, in (semi)residential settings, there is usually a combination of individual and group psychotherapy. The latter utilises specific factors that I have already described and explained in detail in my trilogy on psychodynamic psychiatry. It is essential that both supportive and containing techniques, as well as more classical interpretative techniques, are used. Initially, a safe relationship of trust is established, which is a necessary (but insufficient) condition for the actual psychoanalytic work. There, unconscious loyalties and identifications are worked on, the false self is dismantled, feelings of guilt and compassion with the parental object are explored, and repetitions are identified. Only after their origins have been traced can they be tackled (always with the necessary time and energy), root and branch. Psychoanalysis spins a thread from the tangle, which the patient can use to free themselves from the labyrinth of their unconscious and history.

In conclusion, we can say that parentification in the context of alcohol poses a serious threat to psychosocial development with broad and lasting psychological impact. From a psychoanalytical point of view, the inner world of ACA is distorted by family dynamics that scar the ego strength, object relations, and the self. Long-term psychotherapeutic work attempts to deconstruct these dynamics, restore appropriate boundaries and relationships, help develop true subjectivity, and promote the development of a more integrated and independent self. In this chapter, epidemiology and empirical research were brought into dialogue with psychodynamics and psychogenesis. Psychoanalysis expresses the grammar of what lies beneath the figures: the inadequate parental container, the introjected symptom, the role reversal, the crypt, and so on. The figures reveal where the risks lie, and the story that unfolds in psychoanalysis explains how and why this has happened. The encounters in the consulting room aim to break destructive cycles and enable a new beginning in which (often transgenerational) 'inheritance' gives way to mentalisation, symbolisation, and personal desires that can come into their own.

Notes

1 Hope, Barry, and Byrne (2018).
2 Woititz (1983); Wegscheider-Cruse (1989).
3 Velleman and Templeton (2016).
4 Kane et al. (2024); Westman et al. (2022).

5 World Health Organisation (2018).
6 Tedgård, Råstam, and Wirtberg (2019); Schier (2012).
7 Cuijpers, Langendoen, and Bijl (1999).
8 Hope, Barry, and Byrne (2018).
9 Matthys (2000).
10 Bekir et al. (1993).
11 Chase, Deming, and Wells (1998).
12 Kelley et al. (2007).
13 Chase, Deming, and Wells (1998).
14 Pasternak and Schier (2012).
15 Chase, Deming, and Wells (1998); Kelley et al. (2007); Pasternak and Schier (2012); Hicks (2023).
16 Goglia et al. (1992).
17 Hooper and Doehler (2012).
18 Cuijpers, Langendoen, and Bijl (1999).
19 Cuijpers and Bolier (2001).
20 Widom (1993).
21 Burnett et al. (2006).
22 Cleaver, Unell, and Aldgate (2011).
23 Barnard and Barlow (2003, p. 48).
24 Hoste (2010).
25 Park and Schepp (2015).
26 Goglia et al. (1992).
27 I have discussed this extensively before (Kinet, 2006).
28 Koob and Volkow (2016).
29 Fonagy and Target (2003).
30 Verhaeghe (2002).
31 Bion (1970, p. 15).
32 Rado (1926).
33 Masson (1985).
34 Freud (1905).
35 Freud (1905).
36 Freud (1917).
37 Verheul and van den Brink (1999).
38 Fenichel (1946, p. 376, 510–511).
39 Kohut (1971).
40 Glover (1932).
41 Rosenfeld (1960).
42 Bion (1962b).
43 Bion (1965).
44 McDougall (1989).
45 Bourdellon (2004, p. 448).
46 Aronovsky (2000).
47 Bourdellon (2004, p. 442).
48 '*La jouissance est interdite* à *qui parle comme tel*' (Lacan, 1966, p. 838).
49 Loose (2002, p. 57).
50 Lacan (1991, p. 17).
51 Holzer (1983–1985).
52 Braunstein (1992, p. 257).
53 Bergeret (1981).
54 Monjauze (2000, 2004).
55 Monjauze (2000).

56 Monjauze (2004).
57 Stuyt (2007).
58 Monjauze (2004).
59 Vanheule and Verhaeghe (2004).
60 Vandermeeren (2004).
61 Kornaszewska-Polak (2019).
62 See later chapters discussing this concept in Ferenczi and Anna Freud.
63 Kreisman and Straus (1989).
64 Fischer and Crawford (1992).
65 Hyysalo et al. (2022).
66 Priel and Besser (2001).
67 El-Guebaly, Offord, and Boyle (1993); Kornaszewska-Polak (2019).
68 Domenico and Windle (1993).
69 Hinshelwood (1991).
70 Fairbairn (1943).
71 Klein (1940).
72 Bohm and Esser (2023); Kuppens et al. (2020).
73 Freud (1921).
74 Ferenczi (1932).
75 Lacan (2005).
76 Bion (1962a, p 309). 'Where the mother's alpha-function is absent, the infant is left with beta-elements which accumulate as nameless dread: a state of fear that cannot be thought about, only acted upon or projected into the object.'
77 Mardani et al. (2023).
78 'Incorporation is the construction within the ego of a secret tomb, a crypt that contains the lost object and the unsaid' (Abraham and Torok, 1972, p. 127).
79 Puchol-Martínez, Puchol-Ferrándiz, and Castellano-Tejedor (2023).
80 Rapa et al. (2025).
81 Van Schoors et al. (2023).

References

Abraham, N., and Torok, M. (eds) (1972). Deuil ou mélancolie: Introjection et incorporation, l'introject et le fantôme. *L'écorce et le noyau* (pp. 125–164). Paris: Flammarion.

Aronovsky, D. (Director) (2000). *Requiem for a Dream*. Universal Pictures.

Barnard, M., and Barlow, J. (2003). Discovering parental drug dependence: silence and disclosure 1. *Children and Society*, 17(1), 45–56. doi:10.1002/chi.727

Bekir, P., McLellan, T., Childress, A. R., and Gariti, P. (1993). Role reversals in families of substance misusers: A trans-generational phenomenon. *International Journal of the Addictions*, 28(7), 613–630.

Bergeret, J. (1981). *Le psychanalyse à l'écoute du toxicomane*. Paris: Dunod.

Bion, W. R. (1962a). A theory of thinking. *International Journal of Psycho-Analysis*, 43, 306–310.

Bion, W. R. (1962b). *Learning from Experience*. London: Heinemann.

Bion, W.R. (1965). *Transformations*. London: Heinemann.

Bion, W. R. (1970). *Attention and Interpretation*. London: Karnac.

Bohm, M. K., and Esser, M. B. (2023). Associations between parental drinking and alcohol use among their adolescent children: findings from a National Survey of

United States Parent-Child Dyads. *Journal of Adolescent Health*, 73(5), 961–964. doi:10.1016/j.jadohealth.2023.05.028

Bourdellon, G. (2004). Engagement dans le désir ou engouffrement dans la dépendance. *Revue Française de Psychanalyse*, LXVIII, 441–457.

Braunstein, N. (1992). *La jouissance. Un concept Lacanien*. Paris: Point hors ligne.

Burnett, G., Jones, R. A., Bliwise, N. G., and Ross, L. T. (2006). *Family unpredictability, parental alcoholism, and the development of parentification. American Journal of Family Therapy*, 34 (3), 181–189. doi:10.1080/01926180600550437

Chase, N. D., Deming, M. P. and Wells, M. C. (1998). Parentification, parental alcoholism, and academic status among young adults, *American Journal of Family Therapy*, 26, 105–114. doi:10.1080/01926189808251091

Cleaver, H., Unell, I., and Aldgate, J. (2011). *Children's Needs–Parenting Capacity: Child Abuse, Parental Mental Illness, Learning Disability, Substance Misuse and Domestic Violence* (2nd ed.). London: The Stationery Office.

Cuijpers P., Langendoen, Y. and Bijl R. V. (1999). Psychiatric disorders in adult children of problem drinkers: prevalence, first onset and comparison with other risk factors. *Addiction*, 94 (10), 1489–1498. doi:10.1046/j.1360-0443.1999.941014895.x

Cuijpers, P. and Bolier L. (2001). *Drankjewel: Een zelfhulpgids voor volwassen kinderen van probleemdrinkers*. Utrecht: Trimbos-Instituut.

Domenico, D., and Windle, M. (1993). Parental alcoholism and adult female offspring: Negative life events, personal resources, depression, and parenting. *Journal of Marriage and the Family*, 55 (2), 325–335.

El-Guebaly, N., Offord, D. R., and Boyle, M. H. (1993). Individual and familial characteristics of children of alcoholics. *The Canadian Journal of Psychiatry*, 38 (7), 472–480.

Fairbairn, W. R. D. (1943). The repression and the return of bad objects. In: *Psychoanalytic Studies of the Personality*. London: Tavistock, 1952, 59–81.

Fenichel, O. (1946) *The Psychoanalytic Theory of the Neuroses*. New York: Norton, 510–511.

Ferenczi, S. (1932). *The Clinical Diary of Sándor Ferenczi* (M. Balint, ed.; M. Dupont, trans.). Cambridge, MA: Harvard University Press, 1988.

Fischer, J. L., and Crawford, D. W. (1992). Codependence and parenting styles. *Family Relations*, 41 (2), 204–210.

Fonagy, P., and Target, M. (2003). *Psychoanalytic Theories: Perspectives from Developmental Psychopathology*. London: Whurr.

Freud, S. (1905). Three essays on the theory of sexuality. In J. Strachey (ed. and trans.), *S. E.* (Vol. 7, pp. 125–245). London: Hogarth, 1953.

Freud, S. (1917). Introductory lectures on psycho-analysis (Part III). In *S. E.* (Vol. 16, pp. 243–463). London: Hogarth, 1963.

Freud, S. (1921). Group psychology and the analysis of the ego. In *S. E.* (Vol. 18, pp. 65–143). London: Hogarth, 1955.

Glover, E. (1932). On the etiology of drug addiction. *On the Early Development of the Mind* (pp. 187–215). London: Imago, 1956.

Goglia, L. R., Jurkovic, G. J., Burt, A. M., and Burge-Callaway, K. G. (1992). Generational boundary distortions by adult children of alcoholics: Child-as-parent and child-as-mate. *The American Journal of Family Therapy* 20 (4), 291–299. doi:10.1080/01926189208250899

Hicks, H. R. (2023) Experiences and long-term implications of childhood parentification and parental substance misuse: a scoping review, *McNair Scholars Research Journal*, 26, Article 6. doi:10.32855/2642-2492.1005

Hinshelwood, R. D. (1991). *A Dictionary of Kleinian Thought*. London: Free Association Books.

Holzer, J. (1983–1985). Protect Me from What I Want. LED Sign. *Survival Series.*

Hooper, L. M., and Doehler, K. (2012). Assessing family caregiving: A comparison of three retrospective parentification measures. *Journal of Marital and Family Therapy*, 38 (4), 653–666. doi:10.1111/j.1752-0606.2011.00258.x

Hope, A., Barry, J., and Byrne, S. (2018). *The Untold Story: Harms Experienced in the Irish Population Due to Others' Drinking*. Dublin: Health Service Executive (HSE).

Hoste, M. (2010) Verslaving: de ideale voedingsbodem voor parentificatie. In: M. Kinet (ed.) *Parentificatie. Als het kind te snel ouder wordt* (pp. 123–146). Antwerpen/Apeldoorn: Garant.

Hyysalo, N., Gastelle, M., and Flykt, M. (2022). Maternal pre-and postnatal substance use and attachment in young children: A systematic review and meta-analysis. *Development and Psychopathology*, 34 (4), 1231–1248. doi:10.1017/S0954579421000134

Kane, K., Westman, J., Gissler, M., Jayaram-Lindström, N., and Franck, J. (2024). Risk of severe mood and anxiety disorders in the adult children of parents with alcohol use disorder: A nationwide cohort study. *Journal of Epidemiology and Community Health*, 78 (7), 444–452. doi:10.1136/jech-2023-221720

Kelley, M. L., French, A., Bountress, K., Keefe, H. A., Schroeder, V., Steer, K., Fals-Stewart, W., and Gumienny, L. (2007). Parentification and family responsibility in the family of origin of adult children of alcoholics. *Addictive Behaviors*, 32 (4), 675–685. doi:10.1016/j.addbeh.2006.06.010

Kinet, M. (2006) Een langgerekte kortsluiting. *Zuchtigheid en afhankelijkheid* (pp. 9–23). Antwerpen-Apeldoorn: Garant.

Klein, M. (1940). Mourning and its relation to manic-depressive states. *Love, Guilt and Reparation and Other Works 1921–1945* (pp. 344–369). London: Virago, 1988.

Kohut, H. (1971). *The Analysis of the Self.* New York: International Universities Press.

Koob, G. F., and Volkow, N. D. (2016). Neurobiology of addiction: A neurocircuitry analysis. *The Lancet Psychiatry*, 3 (8), 760–773. doi:10.1016/S2215-0366(16)00104–00108

Kornaszewska-Polak, M. (2019). Attachment in adult children of alcoholics. *Current Issues in Personality Psychology*, 7 (1), 1–12.

Kreisman, J. J., and Straus, H. (1989). *I Hate You, Don't Leave Me: Understanding the Borderline Personality.* New York: Avon.

Kuppens, S., Moore, S. C., Gross, V., Lowthian, E., and Siddaway, A. P. (2020). The enduring effects of parental alcohol, tobacco, and drug use on child well-being: A multilevel meta-analysis. *Development and psychopathology*, 32 (2), 765–778. doi:10.1017/S0954579419000749

Lacan, J. (1966). *Écrits.* Paris: Seuil.

Lacan, J. (1991). *The Seminar of Jacques Lacan, Book V: The Formations of the Unconscious* (J.-A. Miller, ed.). Cambridge: Polity Press.

Lacan, J. (2005). *Le Séminaire, Livre XXIV: L'insu que sait de l'une-bévue s'aile à mourre (1976–1977)* (J.-A. Miller, ed.). Paris: Seuil.

Loose, R. (2002). *The Subject of Addiction. Psychoanalysis and the Administration of Enjoyment*. London/New York: Karnac.

Mardani, A., Jafari, E., Safari, Y., Khamnian, Z., and Alipour, F. (2023). Challenges in addiction-affected families: A systematic review of qualitative studies. *BMC Public Health*, 23, 989.

Masson, J. M. (ed. and trans.). (1985). *The Complete Letters of Sigmund Freud to Wilhelm Fliess, 1887–1904*. Cambridge, MA: Harvard University Press.

Matthys F. (2000). *Leven met een verslaafde*. Antwerpen-Appeldoorn: Garant.

McDougall, J. (1989). *Les théâtres du corps*. Paris: Gallimard.

Monjauze, M. (2000). *Alcoolisme et processus psychiques*. Paris: Dunod.

Monjauze, M. (2004). L'alcoolisme: entre clivage et effondrement. *Revue Française de Psychanalyse*, 68 (5), 1617–1632.

Park, S., and Schepp, K. G. (2015). A systematic review of research on children of alcoholics: Their inherent resilience and vulnerability. *Journal of Child and Family Studies*, 24 (5), 1222–1231. doi:10.1007/s10826-014-9930-7

Pasternak, A., and Schier, K. (2012). The role reversal in the families of Adult Children of Alcoholics. *Archives of Psychiatry and Psychotherapy*, 14 (3), 51–57.

Priel, B., and Besser, A. (2001). Vulnerability to depression: The contribution of attachment styles and the regulation of self-worth. *Personality and Individual Differences*, 31 (5), 789–801.

Puchol-Martínez, F., Puchol-Ferrándiz, A., and Castellano-Tejedor, C. (2023). Preventive interventions for children and adolescents of parents with mental illness: A systematic review. *Clinical Psychology and Psychotherapy*, 30 (5), 979–997. doi:10.1002/cpp.2850

Rado, S. (1926). The psychic effects of intoxicants: an attempt to evolve a psychoanalytical theory of morbid cravings. *Int. J. Psychoanal.*, XII, 396–413.

Rapa, E., Dodsworth, J., Ntuli, A., Anderson, J., Harper, G., and Stein, A. (2025). 'I don't know what to tell them': Experiences of patients talking about mental illness with children and how clinical teams can help. *Frontiers in Psychology*, 16, 1504130. doi:10.3389/fpsyg.2024.1504130

Rosenfeld, H. (1960). The psychopathology of drug addiction and alcoholism: a critical review of the psychoanalytic literature. *Psychotic States* (pp. 217–252). London: Hogarth Press, 1964.

Schier, K. (2012). The role reversal in the families of adult children of alcoholics. *Archives of Psychiatry and Psychotherapy*, 14 (3), pp. 51–57.

Stuyt, A. (2007). Psychoanalyse en alcoholisme: Michèle Monjauze en haar klinische inzichten. *Tijdschrift voor Psychoanalyse*, 16 (1), 119–134.

Tedgård, E., Råstam, M., and Wirtberg, I. (2019). An upbringing with substance-abusing parents: Experiences of parentification and dysfunctional communication. *NAD Nordic Studies on Alcohol and Drugs*, 36 (3), 223–247. doi:10.1177/1455072518814308

Van Schoors, M., Van Lierde, E., Steeman, K., Verhofstadt, L. L., and Lemmens, G. M. (2023). Protective factors enhancing resilience in children of parents with a mental illness: A systematic review. *Frontiers in Psychology*, 14, 1243784. doi:10.3389/fpsyg.2023.1243784

Vandermeeren, R. (2004). Psychoanalytische reflecties over zelf en object in alcoholisme. *Tijdschrift voor psychoanalyse* 10, 135–147.

Vanheule, S., and Verhaeghe, P. (2004). Narcisme, alcoholisme en tegenoverdracht. *Tijdschrift voor Psychoanalyse*, 10 (2), 133–150.

Velleman, R., and Templeton, L. J. (2016). Impact of parents' substance misuse on children: an update. *BJPsych Advances*, 22 (2), 108–117. doi:10.1192/apt.bp.114.014449

Verhaeghe, P. (2002). *Over normaliteit en andere afwijkingen*. Leuven/Leusden: Acco.

Verheul R., and van den Brink W. (1999). Persoonlijkheidsstoornissen. In: de Jong A., van den Brink W., Ormel J. and Wiersma D. (eds), *Handboek psychiatrische epidemiologie*. Maarsden: Elsevier/de Tijdstroom.

Wegscheider-Cruse, S. (1989). *Another Chance: Hope and Health for the Alcoholic Family*. Palo Alto, CA: Science and Behavior Books.

Westman, J., Jayaram-Lindström, N., Kane, K., Franck, J., and Gissler, M. (2022). Mortality in adult children of parents with alcohol use disorder: A nationwide register study. *European Journal of Epidemiology*, 37 (8), 815–826. doi:10.1007/s10654-022-00883-4

Widom, C. S. (1993). Child abuse and alcohol use and abuse. In: Martin, S. E. (ed.), *Alcohol and Interpersonal Violence: Fostering Multidisciplinary Perspectives* (pp. 291–314). Rockville, MD: National Institute on Alcohol Abuse and Alcoholism.

Woititz, J. G. (1983). *Adult Children of Alcoholics*. Deerfield Beach, FL: Health Communications.

World Health Organisation. (2018). *Global Status Report on Alcohol and Health 2018*. Geneva: WHO.

Chapter 8

Intermezzo III

Parentification: Three Clinical Vignettes

To illustrate the above, I will describe three cases in which alcohol and parentification proved to be decisive causal factors.

Sam is a sporty fifty-something with a high flower power content. He is an only child. His mother was a teacher. She always wanted to do good for everyone and is described as overprotective. His father is a retired labourer. As a boy, he looked up to his father because he was so creative and handy. During his early years, there was a lot of tension and conflict at home as a result of his father's alcohol abuse. When he had been drinking, his father was physically aggressive, threatening, and sometimes injuring his mother, so that she had to flee the house with Sam on several occasions. Sam tried to understand and mediate, feeling constantly caught between his parents. He always felt different from his peers. After all, he had a secret. He had to hide something. Everything was hushed up (largely under pressure from his mother). She suffered in silence but meanwhile maintained appearances. For his part, Sam felt that everything was wrong at home. He never felt like he belonged anywhere and tried anxiously to meet everyone's expectations. His studies came second. His main task was to keep the peace and watch over his home. After studying Latin and mathematics in high school, he obtained only a bachelor's degree. *Only* because he feels he has not been able to fulfil his potential. He worked for a company for a long time but left because it was unsatisfying. 'I expected too much: I want recognition and appreciation.' Since then, he has been working as a municipal employee. He lived with his parents for a long time. He went out a lot and drank excessively. He has wrecked several cars and feels he has had a narrow escape. His relationships have also been difficult. As a child, he was very close to Nicole, a girl from his street who was one year younger. They grew up together. As a teenager, she started dating other boys she knew from school. She confided in Sam about her 'relationships' with them—her crushes and heartbreaks. It hurt because he was secretly in love with her himself and couldn't find a way to express it. However, he still felt special because she continued to see him as her most important support, alongside her friends. As they got older, their contact faded. At college, he met Josephine. They were both somewhat withdrawn and found friendship in each other. She could drink

DOI: 10.4324/9781003645726-8

heavily and was a match for any man. She was a good student and they motivated each other, but she fell in love with the bartender… Years later, Sam started seeking out girls of pleasure. He only met them in hotels. He found that more personal. One girl (Elisa) struck him from the first meeting, and they arranged to meet a second time. They spent the hour just talking, but Sam didn't mind at all; he felt mutual understanding and trust. They continued to see each other, sometimes several times a week, and they talked incessantly. Sam was hopelessly in love, but she was in a relationship. This lasted about a year. In the summer, she went on holiday with her boyfriend, and after that, they didn't meet again, although they did send each other a few text messages. During this period, he sometimes made other appointments with a 'young lady' where intimacy did occur. In the years that followed, he continued to seek out 'girls' regularly. At work, he met Valerie, a female colleague. When he first saw her, something strange came over him. She was new and eager to learn; he shared his professional knowledge with her. One thing led to another, and they quickly became a couple. It was his first 'real' relationship. But Valerie herself struggled with many fears; Sam was happy to be a listening ear. In the relationship, he often took on a supportive role, and later on, a work-related problem was added to the mix. The relationship was under increasing pressure, and they both sought professional help, but that could not save the relationship.

A few weeks after the start of his clinical psychotherapeutic admission, he met someone who could move him again for the first time (Marilyn). It turned out that she was a victim of trafficking and was being terrorised by a pimp. He had deeply emotional conversations with her and made plans to rescue her from the clutches of bad men. Although she received him scantily clad and ready to have sex, he did not feel a strong need for sexual contact. On the contrary, there was a fiery platonic infatuation that made him sing her praises despite flagrant evidence to the contrary. He offered her a great deal of financial support and considered kidnapping her and all her belongings to safer places. She missed her six-year-old son, who had stayed with her parents in her home country. Sam was faced with a closed door several times, but he did not give up. At the end of the year, she was due to return to her homeland and, since it was also her son's birthday, he bought a doctor's kit because the boy wanted to be one when he grew up. Later, she sent a photo of her son proudly wearing the doctor's coat. 'I really enjoyed being with her; we both enjoyed a moment of relaxation and peace, and the way we filled the intimate moments was just right for me.' He no longer wanted to see her on a 'conditional' (paying) basis, but he couldn't bring himself to say so clearly. They did stay in touch by telephone, even for a few years after their last live meeting. At one point, she asked for financial help. Sam suggested a 'normal' meeting, but she refused. She indicated that she was seriously ill. After that, contact faded away.

During his (semi)residential psychotherapy, he became fascinated by a fellow patient, Sofie, who belonged to his treatment group. In his view, she was in a clear state of emotional weakness and avoided any attempt at contact. Over a few months, through the clinic's evening sports activities, trust and respect grew. As he got to know her better, he fell in love, even though he saw no possibility of doing anything about it. Forming relationships was prohibited for therapeutic reasons, and Sofie was in a relationship herself. Nevertheless, over time, she sensed how Sam felt about her, and they had long, intense conversations. The way she treated him and conveyed the message that a relationship was not an option for her increased his respect and affection for her, as well as his conviction that he was indeed still capable of entering into an honest and genuine, deeply human relationship. This year, he has once again fallen passionately in love with someone who is not available. Never before has anyone been able to touch his heart so quickly and so deeply.

In addition to these relationship difficulties, Sam had another important issue. He spent many sessions discussing social problems. The neoliberal altar of More, Faster, and Better was particularly targeted. How the 'little man' in particular is crushed by a capitalist juggernaut. How we are perishing in a crazed economic treadmill, how we are exploiting Mother Earth and sending her to the moon. Much of his free time was spent in an alternative community where sustainable nature management and ecological horticulture prevail. There he met like-minded people who, united and in an atmosphere of emotional openness, rolled up their sleeves (also literally) and got to work. He also devoured all kinds of books that exposed progress and advocated replacing patriarchal madness with a more egalitarian society. He was always very passionate in his arguments, but equally frustrated by the fact that, like David, he always had to bow down to this Goliath. He was constantly on the go, rushing from one place to another to help everyone. Meanwhile, he complained that he took little care of himself. He wanted to travel, go for walks by the sea, and enjoy a nice, extensive dinner at a restaurant, but none of that ever happened. He was tired and wondered where it was all leading. When it came down to it, he was alone and missed having a life partner.

We can never really remember wanting to be the one and only for one or both of our parents, and wanting to eliminate our competitors to achieve that. It's symbolic-imaginary variations on certain themes that contain clues to stereotypes that play out in our lives and are linked to the Oedipus complex. In Sam's case, they imply elements of emotional incest, spousification, and parentification that had led him to a barren, if not dead-end, path in his own life.

Emily is in her late twenties and a physiotherapist. She has been experiencing ups and downs for several years when she comes to see me. She suddenly started crying heavily after what had been a pleasant family moment. Since then, her GP has prescribed her a mild antidepressant. She feels that she is on the wrong path. She describes herself as introverted and hypersensitive. She needs rest because she has too much on her mind. She simply feels 'worn out.' Emily is the youngest of four. According to her, her older brother and sisters are all 'doing well': married with children and professionally on track. She herself started to crash at university, where she suddenly felt very alone. It was all about studying, studying, and more studying because she suffered greatly from procrastination and did all kinds of pointless things except study. During her studies, she also clashed a lot with her supervisors and had difficulty with agreements, rules, and authority. Her mother had gone into psychotherapy and had changed from an often drunk and verbally and sexually uninhibited woman (who, as it later turned out, had a serious history of domestic violence, including sexual violence) to complete abstinence and a much more emotionally balanced and stable demeanour. This ultimately led Emily to seek help herself. After all, she had always valued her independence. She saw herself as a planner and a do-it-yourselfer. She therefore found her 'attacks' of helplessness very difficult to cope with. She did worry a lot. It turned out that she had not had an 'easy childhood.' Her parents did not have a loving relationship. They owned a large clothing store and were constantly busy with it. There were many conflicts in which her mother cried, and her father laughed at her and humiliated her. Emily tried to mediate and comfort her mother. Emily also remembered how she often sat alone in various corners of the shop playing. Not that it bothered her at the time. After all, she felt she had complete freedom.

They never did anything together as a family. She also remembers receiving almost as much attention from some regular customers as from her own parents. Even in primary school, Emily felt different from her classmates. She was a leader, often took the lead, and cared for the underdogs. She was very active outside of school: sports, music school, and art classes. In secondary school, she also felt more mature and responsible. Her parents divorced when she was fifteen. Her brother and sisters had already left home. She stayed with her mother, with whom she had always been very close. For a long time, she seemed unaware of her mother's problems. For example, she thought for a long time that alcohol was just her mother's body odour! After the divorce, she tried to take better care of her mother and interfered in her mother's affairs. Good at maths and biology, she chose her own field of study. During her adolescence, she was not interested in boys. So far, she had only had one short-lived relationship with a young man her age who, like her, was independent, mature and hard-working. He also had a difficult childhood with an alcoholic mother. She could not and did not want to really commit to him, and also had difficulties with sexuality, which she associated with her mother's contradictory mixture of obscene language and behaviour when she was under the influence and a repulsive and disapproving attitude towards men when she was sober.

In her psychotherapy (which only got off the ground in fits and starts), Emily talks about feelings of abandonment and depression that sometimes overwhelm her. She also mentions the fact that she has not developed any discipline, which she associates with a total lack of parental supervision. A striking example is how she always stayed up late, arrived at school in the morning without breakfast, was tired and late, and was then told off. There were no boundaries or structure at home. She therefore feels pedagogically neglected and believes she has learned certain important things in life insufficiently or incorrectly. Above all, her development is very one-sided, characterised by (her words) intellectual hypertrophy and subjective and sexual hypotrophy. There is a pattern of parentification in which she has always watched over the relationship between her parents and her mother's alcohol problem, resulting in an imbalance in her personality and a detrimental impact on both her psychosocial and sexual life and experiences. During her therapeutic process, she realises that she has reached a dead end:

> I suffer from loneliness. I miss love and guidance; I have had to do everything on my own my whole life. I have automatically made the wrong choices. I studied and went to work as was expected of me. Now I want to prioritise other things and focus primarily on my feelings and my relationships.

Naturally, a great deal of attention and care is devoted to development assistance in these areas, not least from the matrix of the therapeutic relationship.

Sharon was in her late twenties when she was admitted for clinical psychotherapy. 'They couldn't cope with me, I couldn't get anything done anymore.' Her mother lives with her, but according to Sharon, they can no longer communicate. Sharon went into a fugue state and ended up many kilometres from her home, completely at her wits' end, on a railway track. Her first words were: 'I didn't have a happy childhood, but I always hid that from everyone.' She had her first breakdown on Christmas Eve a few years earlier:

> I had to leave my parents. I went looking for my own place to live. I am single. I work in education, but I don't have a permanent contract and therefore no job security. I became completely silent. I escaped into babysitting. I worked as a nanny in a family with two children. I spent all my time there. My mother wanted a divorce, but she came to live with me. Shortly afterwards, she had a stroke, which left her paralysed on one side for quite some time. Fortunately, she has largely recovered and currently works part-time as a domestic helper. My father was a labourer but has been on disability for years. After work, he always sat in the pub. We could never do anything right for him. He was always shouting and ranting. I was afraid of him. How will he come home tonight? Father was never involved with or concerned about his children. He always wants to have his way.

To this day, he has no idea how much his family has suffered because of his alcohol problem.

Sharon describes her mother as too well-behaved and too dependent. She had wanted a divorce for ten years and often considered escaping to a refuge. There is a younger sister, Anne, who lives with her father. Anne has always been her father's apple of the eye and favourite. They share a passion for classic cars and often go out together to pursue that hobby. Sharon herself was always fearful, shy, and well-behaved. She was an outsider in class and was often laughed at. Fortunately, during her adolescence, she learned to dance hip-hop and, through dancing and trampoline jumping, found an outlet and had some fun. She was also always very close to her mother and stood by her side. She has never been in love or in a relationship. After all, she wants nothing to do with boys or men. Her father is not exactly an appealing role model, and her mother mainly portrays men as sexual predators. 'Which doesn't mean I'm into women!' She would also be afraid to bring someone home because she is ashamed of both her parents.

Sharon underwent two years of clinical psychotherapy. She had been emotionally overwhelmed for a long time. Every day, she caused drama and commotion in the ward and was very clingy and demanding towards fellow patients and staff. In conversations, however, she was quick to get to the point and expressive. She talked mainly about how her mother had manipulated her in all kinds of ways and how she was barely able to live her own life. Thanks in particular to a different/our motherly environment, we saw her gradually blossom. She had to stand her ground for a long time to get her mother out and into a different home of her own. She combined day therapy with returning to work, started going to parties where she could let loose on the dance floor, and underwent a complete makeover, with her skirts getting shorter and her curls and make-up becoming more prominent. She is currently undergoing fertility treatment as a consciously unmarried mother. 'We'll see if a man comes along sooner or later, but I don't need one for sex.' In the meantime, she rides on the back of her older, married neighbour's motorbike through Flanders, and they enjoy stopping at a terrace here and there.

Chapter 9

Psychoanalytic vs Systemic Approaches

Individual and Family

Every personality can be regarded as a conglomeration of (over)sensitivities. In parents and children, these sensitive strings also work transgenerationally. Not only do attachment patterns (aka basic transmissions) express themselves from one generation to the next, but certain themes also continue to resonate in variations. Parents who were raised to be neat and tidy will, in turn, have children who are either the same or the exact opposite—i.e., sloppy and nonchalant. Prudishness turns into debauchery, intrusive intimacy into aloof detachment. However, with the opposite as a crucial element in character formation, + A and − A are both A. After multiplication, this becomes A^2. Thus, the source of conflict and the stumbling block lie ready between the generations.

Apart from little Hans's father, Freud never worked with patients' families. In this case, too, little Hans was the index patient, and it was his environment that requested treatment for him.[1] Apart from this exception, Freud believes that the analyst should keep the family *out of* the consulting room, just as the surgeon does not allow family members into the operating theatre.[2] This attitude has since characterised most psychoanalytic therapists. They are defensive about what they consider to be unwanted interference in domestic affairs. They advance serious, well-founded arguments, such as the importance of discretion and confidentiality, the security and limitations of an intimate or transitional space, and so on. And isn't psychoanalytic therapy a delicate and extremely invasive operation that ultimately focuses on intrapsychic, if not fantastical, reality?

In psychodynamic child psychotherapy, there is a dividing line between the 'schools' of Anna Freud and Melanie Klein, particularly in terms of their attitude towards the family. The Anna Freudian school draws more on research in child and developmental psychology in its theorising. It is cautious about exploring the unconscious, the Oedipus complex, and transference, and advocates a more educational and development-oriented intervention, in which positive transference is stimulated and pursued.[3] The Kleinian school draws

DOI: 10.4324/9781003645726-9

primarily on clinical work in the playroom for its theories. Here, (negative) transference is indeed analysed. After all, it is mainly regarded as the externalisation of inner and fantasmatic distorted (partial) objects, which, given its aggressive/destructive content, is very frightening and pathogenic for the child and must be clearly distinguished from the external reality of the real parents.[4] The net result is that the Kleinians prefer to keep the parents out of the picture, while the Anna Freudians try to involve them closely in the treatment. As is so often the case, however, these differences are mainly highlighted in lectures or publications. In practice, they are probably not so significant.

Psychiatry and Family

Informing the family and involving them in the treatment of the patient has become a key issue for most psychiatric disorders. The potentially important contribution that psychoeducation for the family can make to treatment is also increasingly recognised. Thus, the most advanced (because it is also integrated into the programme offering) family work is found in psychosis care and addiction care. However, when more or less in-depth psychotherapy plays a major role in treatment, involving the family is not always obvious for the patient and/or care provider. Nevertheless, this is particularly necessary in the treatment of children and young people who, by definition, are still dependent on their families in one way or another.

On the team's recommendation, systemic/contextual therapy is sometimes initiated by a specially trained team member. This involves family discussions with parents, particularly in adolescent or young adult patients. They often still live in the parental environment and/or are dependent on it. In particular, processes of individuation and sexualisation can be hindered by the family context and can be addressed and/or discussed in this contextual counselling. More generally, the family is, as it is called, '*not uninvolved*' in the development and/or persistence of psychopathology, about which more will be said later. If indicated, this contextual therapist can also provide partner counselling to promote co-evolution or facilitate dialogue and mediation. For more complex and serious problems, however, regular and, above all, family and/or systemic therapists working outside the setting are called upon. Only they can offer the 'impartiality' necessary to help not the individual but the family or partner system as a whole, without institutionalising or perpetuating scapegoating or exclusion phenomena.

In recent decades, increasing importance has been attached to reflective functioning and mentalisation.[5] These contribute to secure attachment and are an excellent protective factor against the onset of serious psychopathology. After all, they increase *resilience*.[6] Even before the official launch of the so-called KOPP programme, our hospital was already working with the children of our patients in several areas.[7] Social workers try to contribute to organising proper, predictable childcare. Day therapy is encouraged as much as possible to make it seem as if the patient is at work during the day, and age-appropriate reading material is provided. In all of this, it is emphasised that maximum emotional maturity, as well as one's own mental health and well-being, is perhaps the best gift that the patient/parent can give to their child(ren).

Psychoanalytical Approaches

The phenomenon of parentification, in which the child is consciously or unconsciously saddled with the responsibility for caring for one of the parents and/or their relationship, can be described as a pathogenic constellation par excellence. It almost always causes serious emotional disruption to the child's personality. It is the beginning of a fatal domino effect, the shock waves of which can spread far and wide in space and time. Various forms of psychological trauma also trigger mechanisms of repetition compulsion that often continue across generations. Psychoeducation of parents and children can help to neutralise such tragic determinisms.

One of the criticisms that systems thinking has of psychoanalysis is that it focuses too much on the why rather than the how. Psychoanalysis is also said to focus too exclusively on the inner world of the individual patient and to regard him or her too much as a closed system. As a result, it is said to underestimate the importance of interactions with the environment in the (continued) existence of psychopathology. In systems thinking, the individual patient is more of a scapegoat—a lightning rod—a symptom carrier of a system that gets away with it. Furthermore, the supposed linear causality of psychoanalysis is also criticised, whereby the search would be for the unconscious impulse and/or infantile trauma. As if for Freud, the secondary gain with its inherent and vicious circular causality did not exist. And does he not constantly emphasise the importance of Nachträglichkeit or posteriority? The French psychoanalyst André Green discusses in detail the difference between natural and mental causality.[8] In the former, the cause is always sought before the effect, while in psychological matters, causality can also play a retroactive role.

In his introduction to *On Normality and Other Disorders*, Paul Verhaeghe clearly characterises the difference between the medical and any psychotherapeutic model.[9] On the one hand, he gives the example of a four-year-old boy who comes to the doctor's office with chickenpox. The doctor moves from the specific symptom to the general syndrome. What disease is the symptom a sign of? It is an (applied) scientific model with linear causality, in which the cause can always be found (chronologically) before the effect. In contrast, he gives the example of a fifteen-year-old adolescent who joyrides. In this case, the care provider moves from the general to the specific. It turns out that he is an only child, caught between his parents, it always involves a Mercedes (his father's car), and he always ends up in his mother's country, etc. The psychological causality is a layered range of meanings and signifiers. In relation to the symptom, the question is rather what particular meaning and function the symptom has within which relationship and towards whom.[10] The deviant behaviour is therefore always an interpersonal rather than an individual problem. There is always a certain relationship/meaning towards the other person.

Psychoanalysis has a very nuanced view of the aetiopathogenesis of mental disorders. For psychoanalysis, *all* psychopathology is the result of a complex interconnection between three totally different things. There is the reality of drive and predisposition, as well as of fateful or fortuitous coincidence. There is the (safe or unsafe) attachment to the first significant others and the feeling of being affected or gripped by their needs and/or desires. Finally, there is the symbolic order of language and culture, on which each person writes and rewrites their own history. This linguistic aspect of humans as speaking beings creates a division in which biological causalities are not eliminated, but are denatured and, in the broad sense of the word, perverted.[11]

In Lacanian psychoanalysis, it is *even* the Other who calls the shots. Human desire is the desire for/of the Other. The unconscious is the discourse of the Other. Acting out is a question (for translation) addressed to the Other, and so on. But Lacan is not the only one who emphasises the importance of the Other in micro- and macro-culture. For Winnicott, for example, there is *no such thing as a baby* from the outset. He thus lays the foundation for the currently popular *two-person psychology*, with its psychological reality as an essentially joint co-construction.[12]

The object relations school also attaches the utmost importance to the 'objects' that surround us, that ugly technical term for our most important fellow human beings. Our affective relationships are constantly recorded in our psyche and, in turn, determine the lens through which we see others and relate to them. In all these models, the individual is the result of what they have made of their relationship with their environment. Their shadows dance incessantly on the walls of our cave. All relationships with our environment, therefore, have a phantasmal or transference component. For example, even in our relationships with *our current* parents, patterns from the time when they were giants and we were dwarves—the time of fairy tales and caricatures, with their archaic and (technically formulated) partial object transference—continue to play out. With some poetic exaggeration, from a psychoanalytical point of view, we move through a landscape of ghosts throughout our lives.

It is well known that psychoanalysis was the first and, for a long time, the only *talking cure* or conversation therapy. As Freud himself says, since then, many psychotherapies have been simmering on the psychoanalytic fire.[13] Since World War II, however, psychoanalytic forms of treatment have been challenged, mainly by various forms of behavioural therapy. It is a trend that has only been reversed in this millennium by psychoanalysts such as Peter Fonagy and Antony Bateman.[14] They ensured the joyful reintroduction of psychoanalytic treatment in the *Guidelines* of the *American Psychiatric Association* and thus in the world of *evidence-based psychiatry.*[15] Since then, their *Mentalisation-Based Treatment* has been instantly canonised by anyone who calls themselves psychoanalytical: '*Santo Subito*!'

Systemic

In the 1970s and 1980s, systemic therapy also emerged with confidence. Adorned with feathers from various fields, such as General System Theory, cybernetics, mechanics and thermodynamics, biology, epistemology, and communication theory, it immediately assumed a truly scientific allure. With such fresh inspiration and a healthy dose of emancipatory thinking, it stormed many a 'classical' medical-psychiatric or static-nosographic bastion. During my training as a psychiatrist, for example, there was a whole group of enthusiasts at the Psychiatric Centre of KU Leuven (Brussels) who were passionate about these promising developments, which led to the establishment of the LIST (Leuven Institute for System Therapy). Eager to learn, as befits an assistant, I devoured not only the works of nosologists such as Emil Kraepelin, Eugen Bleuler, and Kurt Schneider, but also the texts of the family therapy gurus of the time.

Ludwig von Bertalanffy is considered one of the founders of General Systems Theory.[16] As a biologist, he emphasised the open and dynamic nature of living organisms. He prioritised growth, homeostasis and evolution as central phenomena in all living systems and viewed the world primarily in terms of relationships and integration. He was dissatisfied with reductionist explanatory models, which fall short in understanding living organisms. One of the key concepts in systems theory is holism, which was already proposed by Aristotle in his metaphysics. The whole is more than the sum of its parts. Biological, chemical, social, economic, mental, linguistic factors, etc., do not work cumulatively in contemporary terms, but produce emergence.

Given that this book examines parentification from a psychoanalytical perspective, I will limit myself to an outline of my encounters with various forms of systemic therapy. In Leuven, the Californian group from Palo Alto was particularly popular: they inaugurated a communicative and systemic form of family and relationship therapy that emphasises interaction patterns, meanings, and the role of language and paradox. First, there was Gregory Bateson, a key figure in Palo Alto. He introduced systemic thinking, cybernetics, and communication theory into psychiatry and is best known for the concept of the double bind. This concerns communication patterns in families, which, according to him, could play a role in the development of psychosis. As such, it is outdated, but it remains a valid concept in family therapy to this day. It refers to a paradoxical 'trap' in communication, in which a family member receives contradictory messages and has no way out or opportunity to discuss them.[17] Paul Watzlawick was also inspired by communication theory. He formulated a number of its axioms (e.g., you cannot not communicate, or the difference between the content level and the relationship level) and focused on interaction patterns and the joint construction of reality. Together with colleagues, he developed a short-term strategic family therapy.[18] Don Jackson was also part of the Palo Alto group. He founded the Mental Research Institute and introduced the concept of homeostasis into family interactions.[19] Parallel to the Palo Alto group, developments were taking place in Milan with former psychoanalyst Mara Selvini-Palazzoli, who founded Italy's first family therapy centre. She worked with anorexia patients and their families and also made use of paradoxes and counter-paradoxes. She focused primarily on families with anorexia and psychotic problems.[20] It is questionable if this kind of systemic therapy is compatible with a psychoanalytical approach. This seems to be more the case with figures such as Nathan Ackerman and Murray Bowen, who were initially trained in and indebted to psychoanalysis. Ackerman is often considered the father of family therapy. He combined psychoanalytic thinking with systemic insights and founded the Ackerman Institute for the Family in New York, where intergenerational transmission and related affective psychodynamics are explored and addressed.[21] Bowen, on the other hand, developed his own family systems theory with the following core concepts: differentiation of self, multigenerational transmission process, family projection process and, last but not least, triangulation. Triangulation is the involvement of a third person (usually a child) in the tension field of a dyadic relationship, which temporarily stabilises the system but often at the expense of that third family member. Bowen's starting point is that problems often arise from insufficient differentiation in the family system.[22] Salvador Minuchin, Ivan Boszormenyi-Nagy, and Maurizio Andolfi from the first chapter 'operate' largely along the same lines with their respective structuring and transgenerational approaches. In terms of classics, they can be supplemented by Virginia Satir and Carl Whitaker, both of whom come from an experiential background and whose approaches are also more in line with psychoanalysis. Satir is known for her family sculptures and her focus on family members' self-esteem.[23] Whitaker is best known for his confrontational, creative style, which emphasises humour and imagery. It is a form of therapy based more on art and encounter than on any particular technique.[24]

In recent decades, family therapy has evolved primarily toward postmodern, narrative, and/or attachment theories. In these latter movements, the directive or manipulative family therapy techniques often criticised (e.g. by psychoanalysts) are being replaced by a more 'humble' attitude on the part of the therapist, who explores, discusses, negotiates, etc. on a more equal footing. A number of recent authors from the Anglo-Saxon world are currently leading the way. Susan M. Johnson, for example, is the founder of Emotion Focused Therapy (EFT) for couples and families. She combines attachment theory with systemic therapy and focuses on emotional connection, security, and corrective experiences in family relationships.[25] In line with the psychoanalytic approach, Eia Asen and Peter Fonagy represent mentalisation-based family therapy (MBT-F). The focus is on increasing mentalisation capacity, i. e., understanding your own thoughts, feelings, and intentions, as well as those of other family members.[26] For the sake of completeness, I would like to mention Else-Marie van den Eerenbeemt from the Dutch-language literature, who made scientific insights into family patterns, intergenerational loyalties, and hidden intrafamilial dynamics accessible to a wider audience.[27] Last but not least, I conclude with my compatriot Peter Rober, who focuses primarily on what goes on in the mind and heart of the family therapist. Therapeutic impasses are understood not least as a paralysis of the therapist's 'inner conversation.'[28] Rober talks about three ways of listening in family therapy: with the ears (the narrative layer), with the eyes (non-verbal signals, body language, emotions) and with the heart (what is evoked in the therapist). Listening is not easy or automatic; it requires an attitude of not knowing, curiosity, and openness. In the therapeutic relationship, this implies an ethical attitude: not primarily gathering information, but showing that the family is being heard and recognised in its intentions and experiences. He warns against an aberration that characterised many first-generation family therapists: despite good intentions, assuming a colonising position in the therapeutic relationship, wanting to force change too quickly, taking control, or 'treating' family members as if they were passive. Rober, on the other hand, encourages an attitude that connects primarily with the suffering and strength of the various family members, rather than discouraging them through external restructuring.[29]

A Possible Discussion

Regardless of their orientation, family therapists each try in their own way to promote change and development in families. They are more interested in how problems persist than why they arise. They focus on repetitive interaction patterns rather than intrapsychic fantasies or impulses. They look more at what is happening between people than at what is happening within them. According to Freud, polar bears and whales cannot wage war.[30] After all, they each inhabit a different world. However paradoxical it may sound: '*Pour disputer il faut être d'accord.*' To have a discussion, we need minimal agreement. Well, certainly in their work with children, adolescents, and young adults, psychoanalysts and systemic therapists share the same aim. Regardless of all the theory, we could summarise this as contributing to development aid, and emancipation. If we can all agree on that, at least, we can discuss a great many things.

Systemic thinking does not offer explanations about aetiopathogenesis, it does not shed light on processes of symbolisation, nor does it produce any map of the inner world. Theoretically, however, it has many points of contact with psychoanalysis. For example, it emphasises the importance it attaches to homeostasis as a variant of the Freudian principle of constancy. The same applies to concepts such as equifinality and equipotentiality, in which different initial states lead to the same final state, and vice versa. Many family therapy concepts, such as triangulation, parentification, tangled and loose sand families, family structure and hierarchy, are very recognisable terms in psychoanalysis for describing typical family relationships and/or parent-child configurations. Both recognise that human problems are not purely rational. Both work with patterns (intrapsychic versus interactional). Both are sensitive to transference: in psychoanalysis, as recurring patterns that come alive on stage in and outside of therapy; in systemic therapy, as it appears in interactions, alliances, and triangulations.

When pseudo-balances and morphostatic forces hinder or prevent individual growth, systemic interventions can be useful, necessary, or even indispensable. These do require the cooperation of the other members of the system, which is not self-evident for many hospitalised patients. For example, because they have become completely isolated and/or marginalised, or because there is no longer any possibility of cooperation with the family and other environments. An in-depth and lengthy psychotherapeutic process may then be necessary to acknowledge and process such realities, and to be able to go one's own way.

Families and How to Survive Them. That is the title of the bestseller by Robin Skynner and John Cleese.[31] It is indeed sometimes a real *struggle.* This struggle always requires sweat and tears, sometimes blood, and more rarely, in the full sense of the word, a *struggle for life.* Ultimately, all our patients have to do it themselves, but as far as we are concerned, they do not have to do it alone. Does everything now take place mainly between others or mainly between our ears? The most important question is how or why? Growth and change in our inner, psychological reality should ideally also be realised and/or transformed in our interaction with external reality. Many roads lead to this Rome, but not all. Unfortunately, the only ones who bring us closer to our goal are going uphill against the wind. After all, resistance is also strong in families.

Notes

1 Freud (1909).
2 Freud (1916–1917, p. 602).
3 Anna Freud (1927).
4 Klein (1955).
5 Kinet and Vermote (2005).
6 Fonagy et al. (1994).
7 COMIP: Children Of Mentally Ill Parents.
8 Green (1995).
9 Verhaeghe (2002).
10 Verhaeghe (2002, p. 15).
11 Kinet (2006, pp. 41–47).
12 Boerwinkel and Gomperts (2001).
13 Freud (1933, p. 82).
14 Bateman and Fonagy (2004).

15 American Psychiatric Association (2001).
16 Von Bertalanffy (1968).
17 Bateson (1972).
18 Watzlawick, Beavin, and Jackson (1967).
19 Jackson (1965).
20 Selvini-Palazzoli et al. (1980).
21 Ackerman (1958).
22 Bowen (1978).
23 Satir (1967).
24 Whitaker and Bumberry (1988).
25 Johnson (2019).
26 Asen and Fonagy (2017).
27 Van den Eerenbeemt (2016).
28 'The therapist's inner conversation is described as a negotiation between the self of the therapist and his role … therapeutic impasse is conceptualised as a paralysis of the circle of meaning and of the therapist's inner conversation' (Rober 1999, p 209).
29 Rober (2024).
30 Freud (1916–1917, p 580).
31 Skynner and Cleese (1986).

References

Ackerman, N. W. (1958). *The Psychodynamics of Family Life: Diagnosis and Treatment of Family Relationships.* New York: Basic Books.

American Psychiatric Association. (2001). Practice guidelines for the treatment of patients with borderline personality disorder. *Am. J. Psychiatry*, 158, 1–52.

Asen, E., and Fonagy, P. (2017). *Mentalization-Based Treatment for Families.* New York: Guilford.

Bateman, A. and Fonagy, P. (2004). *Psychotherapy for Borderline Personality Disorder. Mentalization Based Treatment*. London: Oxford University Press.

Bateson, G. (1972). *Steps to an Ecology of Mind.* Oxford, UK: Chandler.

Boerwinkel, A. R., and Gomperts, W. J. (2001). *Alleen en met z'n tweeën. One- en two-person psychologie in de psychoanalyse.* Assen: Van Gorcum.

Bowen, M. (1978). *Family Therapy in Clinical Practice.* New York: Jason Aronson.

Fonagy, P., Steele, M., Steele, H., Higgitt, A. and Target, M. (1994). The theory and practice of resilience. *Journal of Child Psychology and Psychiatry*, 15, 231–257. doi:10.1111/j.1469-7610.1994.tb01160.x

Freud, A. (1927). Four lectures on child analysis. In: *The Writings of Anna Freud* (Vol. I). New York: International Universities Press, 1974.

Freud, S. (1909). De familieroman van de neuroticus. In *Werken* (Vol. 4, pp. 547–550). Amsterdam: Boom, 2006.

Freud, S. (1916–1917). Colleges inleiding tot de psychoanalyse. In *Werken* (Vol. 7, pp. 211–613). Amsterdam: Boom, 2006.

Freud, S. (1933). Colleges inleiding tot de psychoanalyse – Nieuwe reeks. In *Werken* (Vol. 10, pp. 79–232). Amsterdam: Boom, 2006.

Green, A. (1995). *La causalité psychique. Entre nature et culture.* Paris: Odile Jacob.

Johnson, S. M. (2019). *Attachment Theory in Practice: Emotionally Focused Therapy (EFT) with Individuals, Couples, and Families.* New York: Guilford.

Jackson, D. D. (1965). The study of the family. *Family Process*, 4 (1), 1–20.

Kinet, M. and Vermote, R. (eds) (2005). *Mentalisatie*. Antwerpen/Apeldoorn: Garant.
Kinet, M. (2006). *Freud & Co in de psychiatrie. Klinisch-psychotherapeutisch perspectief.* Antwerpen/Apeldoorn: Garant.
Klein, M. (1955). The psycho-analytic play technique: Its history and significance. In *Envy and Gratitude and Other Works 1946–1963* (pp. 122–140). London: Virago, 1988.
Satir, V. (1967). *Conjoint Family Therapy: A Guide to Theory and Technique*. Palo Alto, CA: Science and Behavior Books.
Rober, P. (1999). The therapist's inner conversation in family therapy practice: Some ideas about the self of the therapist, therapeutic impasse, and the process of reflection. *Family Process*, 38 (2), 209.
Rober, P. (2024). *Becoming an Effective Family Therapist: Research, Practice, and Case Stories*. London/New York: Routledge.
Selvini Palazzoli, M., Boscolo, L., Cecchin, G., and Prata, G. (1980). Hypothesizing—circularity—neutrality: Three guidelines for the conductor of the session. *Family Process*, 19 (1), 3–12.
Skynner, R. and Cleese, J. (1986). *Families and How to Survive them*. London: Oxford University Press.
Van den Eerenbeemt, E.-M. (2016). *Door het oog van de familie*. Amsterdam: Balans.
Verhaeghe, P. (2002). *Over normaliteit en andere afwijkingen*. Leuven/Leusden: Acco.
Von Bertalanffy, L. (1968). *General System Theory*. New York: Braziller.
Watzlawick, P., Beavin, J. H., and Jackson, D. D. (1967). *Pragmatics of Human Communication: A Study of Interactional Patterns, Pathologies, and Paradoxes*. New York: Norton.
Whitaker, C. A., and Bumberry, W. M. (1988). *Dancing with the Family: A Symbolic-Experiential Approach*. New York: Brunner/Mazel.

Chapter 10

Intermezzo IV

A Family Portrait of Parentification

A psychiatrist trained in both systemic and psychoanalytic approaches discussed with me during his supervision the experiences of a broken family and its members, whom he and his colleagues had followed closely or from a distance for many years. This provides an exceptionally broad perspective from which to clinically describe (components of) parentification. I will limit myself to a helicopter perspective and a skeletal emotional framework; the reader can flesh it out for themselves.

The family's parents are both architects. Mother Sara is the middle of three daughters and has always felt a bit caught between two stools, left out. Her father was also an architect. He was very successful professionally, and his career took him to various foreign countries, where Sara's family always led a luxurious life with domestic staff. However, her father was an alcoholic and physically and emotionally abusive towards his wife and children, so Sara's mother eventually left and fled with her three children. She found permanent shelter on her own floor in the spacious home of her older sister, Jennifer: all in all, five women ended up under one roof.

Sara's mother never worked and lived comfortably thanks to an inheritance from her father, a renowned painter. In the meantime, she produced some children's literature. As a child, Sara suffered greatly from family tensions, the loss of her father (with whom she sporadically experienced warm and intimate moments that she continued to cherish), and a feeling of displacement. She has had depressive tendencies since childhood, and during her adolescence, she first developed alcohol abuse and later abused psychostimulants, which she used as appetite suppressants to combat obesity. Despite her sophisticated and artistic façade, she has low self-esteem, a great need for positive reinforcement, and is emotionally unstable, mainly because abandonment anxiety, anger, and depression are constantly lurking. She has worked at various architectural firms throughout her career but was repeatedly dismissed for frequent illness-related absences. In recent years, she has had her own firm, which is operating at a low level.

Father Tom is the eldest of two sons. He comes from a loving home with two modest, hard-working parents who worked their way up from the lower

DOI: 10.4324/9781003645726-10

middle class. They were very class-conscious because Tom, as an excellent student, was often invited by 'richer' friends, but his parents did not allow this because of the status difference. Tom himself was given the opportunity for social advancement by his parents, and thanks to his studies and student life, he was able to broaden his socio-cultural horizons considerably. He worked for decades in the same agency, where he rose to the position of co-manager. He is now highly respected in his field.

Tom and Sara met during their student days. In Sara's eyes, Tom was a handsome, sensitive but also dreamy young man. He wanted to study the same subject as Sara's father, bore some physical resemblance to him, and she was charmed by his artistic sensibility and interest. In Tom's eyes, Sara had something of Our Lady of Sorrows about her. He was also impressed by her (in his eyes) high society background. From the beginning, he had noticed her alcohol problem and depressive tendencies, but he looked up to her because of a tragedy and grandeur that, in a sense, both fascinated and impressed him. Their relationship lasted throughout their further education (more than ten years in total) and culminated (after a brief break with other partners during internships in different parts of the country) in a marriage, which was probably motivated more by fear of separation than by desire on both sides.

The start of their professional careers and the birth of their two children (Jane and Henry) led to a truly mature life, but shortly after Henry's birth, Tom fell head over heels in love with a younger female colleague who seemed to him a healthy, cheerful, and uncomplicated live wire. A whole period of comings and goings followed, culminating in a difficult and painful divorce for both parties, with Sara left hurt and abandoned, and Tom's life taking a happier and more joyful turn with Helen. After some acrimonious disputes, Sara and Tom divorced by mutual consent after three years. A year later, Tom and Helen were married. After the divorce, both children stayed with their mother, with a slightly extended version of the classic visiting arrangement with Tom. He paid (mainly out of guilt for his infidelity and so that their mother could maintain their high standard of living) the equivalent of a month's salary in child support, and all these agreements were correctly complied with by both parties in the following years. However, the children lived in two completely different worlds. According to Tom, they had a say in everything at Sara's, were involved in all the household chores, had few boundaries and were (literally) pampered more than was good for them. With Tom and Helen, there were more laws, rules, structure, and regularity. To Tom, they seemed to undergo a complete transformation after each stay with their mother, alternately subject to regressive versus progressive forces. It took him several days each time to 'normalise' the children, which he believed led to a 'zigzag' that would characterise their later lives. Sara was annoyed by Helen's influence on the children's manners and clothing, as well as by Helen's overly maternal attitude towards them. She also portrayed Tom as a controlling, authoritarian figure whom the children had to follow.

During the exchanges, Tom often noticed that Sara was under the influence of alcohol. She had a succession of partners. Occasionally, he heard from the children about arguments and conflicts. One of the partners contacted him in writing (in a letter bearing a number of respectable and unmistakable professional titles) because of Sara's extreme alcohol consumption. How the children repeatedly had to help her undress, ended up in bed with her, were left unattended and unprotected, and so on. He was mobilised to take the necessary action as a father. Meanwhile, there were also more and more irregularities in the visiting arrangements, with Tom (who was always responsible for transport to and from) repeatedly finding himself facing a closed door, even when Sara was indeed at home with the children. When Sara finally checked herself into rehabilitation summer holidays and, given that both parents lived far apart, Tom took the children with him and enrolled them in a school in his place of residence. He had recently become the father of a daughter, Suzy, so he and Helen took all three children into their care and moved from a flat to a more spacious house with a garden.

At the beginning of that school year, Sara and her new partner, Bruno, burst into the school building to take the children away. Bruno was initially one of Sara's patients. He is a few years younger. Although unqualified, he presents himself as a manager, but has been unemployed for years and has been repeatedly called a fantasist by Henry. He has two sons from a previous marriage, both of whom have been admitted to psychiatric care several times, one for (allegedly borderline) personality difficulties, the other for drug addiction. The management was immediately alarmed by the smell of alcohol on the couple and their erratic behaviour; the police were notified, and the youth court prosecutor was called in. After questioning all those involved and the children, it was decided in an emergency hearing that the children would remain with their father and that Sara would only be allowed limited visiting rights (in the presence of a trusted third party). A 'quiet' period followed as long as 'the case' remained under the supervision of the juvenile court. However, when this was dropped to make way for further civil proceedings, situations involving alcohol and intrafamily conflicts soon arose again. After years of legal proceedings (both in the first instance and on appeal, and after the intervention of various judicial assistants and experts), the residence arrangement with the father was confirmed. At first, both children seemed to be doing well at school and socially while living with their father. Within the multidisciplinary team of a Centre for Mental Health (CMH), both received individual psychotherapeutic counselling, and there were regular meetings with each parent separately. One of the experts involved in the legal proceedings described both children as 'mentally healthy' during that period. In the meantime, Sara and Bruno had a son, George. Sara tried to win over the children and bond with them with George's help. She turned to both Jane and

Henry for emotional support and for help with family or financial issues. It was only later that Tom discovered that Jane was meeting with her mother, Sara, 'behind his back.' After her consultations at the CMH, and instead of going to the academy Helen had enrolled her in (at her own request), they went out for cake together. From one day to the next, Jane moved in with her mother after school without saying goodbye to her father's family or her half-sister. This had been carefully planned and prepared with her mother, Sara. Shortly afterwards, Henry joined Jane. Sara and Bruno were triumphant because they had finally succeeded in taking the children away. Tom and Helen (and certainly Suzy) were devastated and in despair. As was to be expected and predictable, however, major problems immediately arose again with their mother: Sara and Bruno's drinking and (as a result) conflicts with the necessary noise. During that period, Tom received several voice messages from Jane, crying, with domestic turmoil clearly audible in the background. After a few months, Jane fled (with Sara's permission) to her former foster mother because, apparently, anything was 'better' than returning to her father's family. Because the abuses continued despite this, the youth court was once again called in (after consultation between Tom and the foster mother). After consultations and discussions, Jane was first placed in care, and the childminder was appointed her foster mother, while Henry was placed in a boarding school. Subsequently, Jane and Henry were reassigned to their father by the new youth court. Jane remained at boarding school because a full return to her father's family was considered unfeasible for all involved. Henry returned to live with his father as a day pupil but withdrew to his room more than before. He had a number of other after-effects. He started using cannabis, was found sitting on park benches like a stoned hippie and was expelled from the gymnastics club for insubordination. He had to leave a holiday camp because he had arranged to meet his girlfriend there, even though this was not allowed. Tom immediately took Henry to the school management when Helen found bags of cannabis in his room. Jane's school results were significantly lower than before her disappearance. She was negligent with her schoolwork and also neglected administrative matters.

After the last intervention by the youth court (and under further supervision until they both reached the age of majority), there were no further irregularities regarding residence or visitation arrangements. Jane was able to finish secondary school (despite periods of unauthorised absences when she was staying with her mother and despite several resits and summer assignments), and Henry (after several years of slacking off and sporadic cannabis use) even graduated at the top of his class. Although their father, Tom, continued to pay all the costs of education and living expenses for both children until they both graduated from university, Jane and Henry hardly ever visited him during their higher education. However, they often spent their weekends and free time with their mother and her friends. With Sara, Bruno, and his two children (both on drugs) more often intoxicated than sober, there was a light-hearted and dreamy atmosphere characterised by *la bohème* and the necessary *flou artistique.* In Sara's eyes, however, Tom and Helen were haughty, materialistic, and narrow-minded bourgeois who had taken advantage of Sara's moments of weakness. In her view, Jane and Henry were her saviours and defenders, and were accorded an important status as key figures and pillars of support. In recent years, the psychiatrist has only had (indirect) information via his colleagues. Jane took ten years to complete her university studies and is now working at degree level. She first had a relationship with a man twenty years her senior who lived on a boat; he and his dog moved in with her, which did not go down well with the landlord, who thought he had rented the studio to a single student. While she was admitted for a year of clinical psychotherapy, she met another man twenty years her senior. He did not finish secondary school, is an unskilled labourer, but presents himself as working in 'the cultural sector' and is the father of an adolescent son for whom he has never paid child support since his divorce, so he has now been ordered by the court to pay off his debts in this regard. They have a daughter together, but Jane is currently going her own way because her partner hardly works and is an alcoholic. Henry completed his university studies within the set period and without any resits, but hardly ever stayed with or visited his father during those years. However, they did go on several trips together to various European cities, during which they talked a lot and expressed themselves (also about emotional issues). He first had a relationship with a classmate from a 'nice family' for several years. He then had a relationship with a girl from a fatherless family. Next, he was with a woman almost thirty years his senior and mother of two children, with whom he travelled several times, and then with his stepbrother's (Bruno's eldest son) drug-addicted ex. After working for several years in a job that matched his university level, he has been working in the hospitality industry at home and abroad for about three years. For the sake of completeness, George has been admitted to rehab several times and has so far tried unsuccessfully to pursue higher education. Suzy and her boyfriend are well on their way to completing a PhD programme.

It is left to the reader to identify the components of split identification and invisible loyalties in this family sketch. There is enmeshment, and the boundaries between the generations seem vague or non-existent. The attachments are incoherent, and elements of spousification and emotional incest are present. Both Jane and Henry bear the marks of parentification associated with a painful cocktail of alcohol and depression, a problematic divorce, and inadequate paternal function.

Chapter 11

Curiously Called. To Cure, to Care

On Calling, Vocation, Profession, and Parentification

Introduction

During my medical studies, I held many student jobs in the hospitality sector. In one of the cafés where I worked, there was a sign behind the bar with the following inscription: 'You don't have to be crazy to work here, but it helps.' Throughout my later career in psychiatry, this sentence often popped into my mind (and with my consent).[1] To this day, I can say with some satisfaction: still crazy after all these years! My profession has always been both a passion and a calling for me. Neither of these occurs in its pure form, of course. As is often the case, they are alloyed with other components. A vocation is sometimes understood as a call to go against nature and devote yourself selflessly to something: a good cause that is not always obvious.[2] A vocation is very similar to passion, but passion comes from within, as something you undergo and of which you are the object, whereas with a vocation, this voice comes from elsewhere. You are seized by a kind of sacred enthusiasm. While passion is transgressive and goes beyond boundaries, vocation sometimes transcends the everyday things of life and is, in that sense, not transgressive but transcendent. Often, in contrast to ambition, vocation is a loss-making activity, but the paradox is that those who feel called have nothing to lose. With a calling, you have an ideal that guides you. With the more primitive ambition, you may be driven more by the desire to *be* ideal. In this context, however, it mainly refers to a *moral* ambition. Instead of salary, prestige, titles, or power, it revolves around the realisation of ideals: impact, a constructive contribution to small and large problems, meaning for others.[3] Every coin has its flip side, and behind such altruistic motives are always less noble components. It is important to know and recognise them, but when this is sufficiently the case, they do not detract from their prosocial content. For many psychotherapists, their calling is ultimately also a curious symptom or a symptom of curiosity.[4] I paraphrase the American short-story writer Dorothy Parker: the only cure for boredom is curiosity; for curiosity there is no cure.

DOI: 10.4324/9781003645726-11

The Choice That Chooses Us

In modern psychology, career choice is usually described as a rational process: you choose a profession based on your interests, talents, and job market opportunities. It is therefore often said that we choose our profession. But perhaps the opposite is true: the profession chooses us. Behind the seemingly conscious process of interests, talents, and market logic lies a complex web of desire, memory, and repetition. What we call a career is often a repetition of earlier emotional scenes: places where we were once recognised, validated, or hurt. Behind every choice lie unconscious motivations, identifications, and patterns of repetition. A profession is never purely an economic activity; it is a compromise between impulse and reality, between the desire of the subject and that of the Big Other. Psychoanalysis considers the choice of profession to be a symbolic inscription of the unconscious. Through their work, the subject seeks not only recognition but also a place within the symbolic order, where old inner conflicts are re-enacted. Psychoanalysis invites us to listen to that undercurrent. It hears in every career choice the echo of a childish dialogue: who must I be to be loved?

Chiara Staal argues that the unconscious determinants of people's career choices can be traced back to our internalised image of the self, the other—usually the parent or caregiver—and the emotional relationship between the two. The choice of a particular career path enables the individual to repeat important childhood experiences, fulfil unmet needs or achieve certain career goals, professional patterns, and expectations from their family of origin.[5]

This chapter examines how classical psychoanalysts (such as Freud, Ferenczi, Klein, Winnicott, Bion, and Lacan) understand career choice as repetition and symbolic compromise formation. Why does Freud call some professions impossible? What is the difference between vocation, the vocational, and the professional? It zooms in on the decision to choose psychological counselling, where personal wounds can carry particular weight. These three layers overlap, showing how work, desire, and subjective vulnerability are intertwined. Finally, the figure of the parentified therapist is discussed, in which the theme of the wounded healer takes on a more specific form.

Freud: Repetition

Sigmund Freud pointed out in one of his technical writings that people tend to repeat past relational patterns rather than remember or process them. He describes how people tend to recreate their past in the present, not by choice but involuntarily or out of necessity.[6] Action replaces insight. This urge to repeat is also expressed in the choice of a profession: you seek out situations that resonate with the original object relations that are being replayed. The doctor who tries to save a sick mother, the lawyer who wants to emulate his father's authority, the teacher who seeks the love he lacked as a child from his audience, or the artist who seeks the affirmation he once lacked. They all stage an earlier scenario, turning their professional lives into a theatre of transference. The latter, therefore, involves an unconscious attempt to bring an old conflict to a better conclusion. In addition to this rather 'benign' repetition, there is also his (more demonic or diabolical) concept of the *compulsion to repeat*, in which particularly painful past experiences are brought to life on stage.[7] Dysfunctional patterns of, for example, loss or trauma can occur in a fruitless attempt to process or master them. In that case, the repetition is caused by a primitive psychological need to bind fear and thus master it. In contemporary attachment theory, this phenomenon is regarded as a return to unresolved inner object relations because, paradoxically, they feel safer or more familiar.[8] A bit like someone born in Siberia who, despite its blatant inhospitableness, may experience homesickness for Siberia. Neuropsychoanalytically, it is about free energy that needs to be bound through predictive coding, and about incentive salience and increased arousal that continue to determine the brain's default mode (more than we would like in that case).[9] This phenomenon presents the patient with major psychotherapeutic challenges because they remain, as it were, a prisoner of inappropriate relationships or situations and seems unable to learn the right lessons from them or break out of them. The aim of the treatment is to break the vicious circles of unconscious repetition through awareness and memory.[10] Underlying fears and unmet needs are at the root of perceived (inter)actions, and only by understanding them can the patient move from a passive victim to the author of his own history. I refer to a memorable one-liner by Vincent de Gaulejac: *l'homme est le produit d'une histoire dont il cherche à devenir le sujet.*[11]

Freud: Sublimation

In Freudian metapsychology, sublimation is both important and, to this day, enigmatic. It is said to underlie a number of human idiosyncrasies, if not to highlight them. Artistic creation and scientific research (or more broadly: all intellectual activity and cultural production) owe their existence to it. After all, they originate from the same energy that animates our most primitive sexual and aggressive drives. True to its etymology, it is a form of alchemy that transforms the lead of essentially animalistic impulses into the gold of civilisation. In their famous psychoanalytical dictionary, Laplanche and Pontalis refer to sublimation as 'one of the most elusive concepts in psychoanalytic theory.'[12]

As such, the word sublimation first appeared in 1897 in a letter to Wilhelm Fliess,[13] but it was not until Freud's Three Essays on the Theory of Sexuality that it was first developed theoretically.[14] The sexual drives he describes in it are extremely vivid. Their purpose can also be changed. In sublimation, for example, the sexual drive is 'turned to a new aim and, in particular, to an aim no longer sexual but socially valued.'[15]

In his economic model of the human mind, Freud initially prioritised the distribution and transformation of libido. From this perspective, sublimation represents an ideal solution to the tension between instinct and society. In contrast to repression (which dams up energy and can lead to symptoms in the form of the veiled return of the repressed), sublimation channels energy into civilised and even appreciated products of civilisation. In this context, Freud also refers to a desexualisation of the drive.[16] His sublimation 'is an especially conspicuous feature of cultural development; it is what makes it possible for higher psychical activities, scientific, artistic or ideological, to play such an important part in civilised life.'[17]

Freud also described labour as a form of sublimation: a socially accepted channel in which instinctual energies find symbolic expression in socially desirable behaviour.[18] The instinct seeks a way, and society gives it form. In work, desire finds a temporary home. Yet labour remains restless: it conceals a hunger that no wage can satisfy. Sublimation may tame the drive, but it preserves its energy. It does not mean healing because, as a cultural detour, it is a compromise. Passion continues to ferment under the cloak of the profession, which, on the other hand, allows aggressive or erotic impulses to find symbolic expression.

From the perspective described so far, career choice becomes a moral and existential issue. It tells us something about how we deal with our shortcomings, how we try to tame or transform them. The psychoanalytical view shifts the question from 'What do I want to become?' to 'What in me desires to be repeated?' After all, work is not only productive but also libidinally charged. Psychoanalysis teaches us that we do not freely choose what we 'become,' but that we choose based on our unconscious structure. Career choice is thus an attempt at self-realisation and self-control: a way of organising and symbolising our instinctual life. It is therefore not a coincidence, but a compromise between unconscious desire and the demands of reality. The choice of a profession reveals the subject's place in relation to their drives and to the Big Other. It can be read as a repetition, but also as an opportunity for transformation: in this re-enactment of the old scenario, something new can emerge.

Freud: Impossibility

Freud later added another insight to all this: certain professions confront people directly with the psyche or unconscious of others. In his essay *Analysis Terminable and Interminable*,[19] he therefore called three professions 'impossible': educating, governing, and analysing. By this, he did not mean that these tasks are impossible to perform, but that they can never be (completely) successful. They confront people with the limits inherent to psychological life and to living together. They are impossible because they work with human subjectivity: capricious, ambivalent, and unpredictable. In education, politics, and therapy, we always encounter resistance, transference and—with the unconscious—the limits of malleability. This is precisely where their ethical dimension lies: one can only act by taking this failure into account.

In education, the teacher stands in front of the class. Before him are rows of desks full of eyes, each child an enigma, each ear a different rhythm. He writes words on the board but knows that no chalk can determine the future. His lesson falls apart as soon as the bell rings. Yet he continues to speak, because silence would be worse. Education is impossible because the teacher or parent can never fully determine how a child will develop. The child is not merely a recipient of knowledge and norms, but a subject with its own pace, fantasies, and resistance. Freud already recognised this: education is a compromise between instinct and culture. The child learns through identification, but also through resistance. It is precisely the failure of education, the residue that cannot be fitted in, that makes unique subjectivity possible. The impossibility of education is therefore not a shortcoming, but on the contrary, precisely the condition for freedom.

Because of governing, the politician stands behind the lectern. He raises his hand above a crowd that cheers and grumbles. Today, his words promise order; tomorrow, they cause riots. Power slips through his fingers like sand. Yet he continues to give orders, because doing nothing is even more dangerous. Freud also calls governing impossible. Political power seems decisive but is always undermined by the unpredictability of the masses, by resistance, and by unconscious identifications. In his text on mass psychology, Freud shows that leadership is based on identification: the leader embodies the ideal ego.[20] But this mechanism is unstable and can turn into hatred and aggression. The impossibility of governing lies in this structural gap: perfect harmony is impossible. Politics can at best mediate in conflicts, but never satisfy all desires. Distrust of politicians often reflects a failure to recognise this structural shortcoming.

The analyst sits in the consulting room. He says little. He listens to a stream of words that both reveal and conceal. Every truth that presents itself slips away again. Healing is never complete, at best a shift. Yet he continues to listen, because speaking itself is the only chance. Psychoanalysis confronts the subject with their unconscious, but the unconscious is precisely that which resists knowledge. Freud emphasises that every analysis is both finite and infinite: finite, because there must always be a moment of closure; infinite, because there always remains a residue that cannot be analysed or resolved.[21] With a nod to Marcel Duchamp, not only every work of art but every psychoanalysis is 'definitively unfinished.'[22] This impossibility of analysis implies its ethical power: the analyst does not promise a complete cure, but a space where the subject can learn to deal with his lack.

Klein: Depressive Position and Repair

The British object relations school distanced itself from Freud's drive-theoretical views on sublimation in two ways. Both Melanie Klein and Donald

Winnicott shifted the emphasis to relationships with our internal and external objects. For Klein, creativity and cultural achievements are not based on sublimated libido, but rather on an archaic struggle with fear and guilt in what she calls the schizoid-paranoid and depressive position. In the depressive position, the child begins to realise that the beloved (good) and the hated (bad or evil) mother are one and the same. This generates intense fear and guilt about the fantasised attacks that the child has committed in the schizoid-paranoid position. The child desperately wants to repair the damage done. For Klein, this reparative urge is the true source of creativity and sublimation. In *Envy and Gratitude*, she writes: 'The desire to make reparation… is, in my view, a fundamental factor in the creative process and sublimation in general.'[23] Painting, writing, or building are a matter of repairing damage. Sublimation is not an economic or alchemical transformation of energy, but a more symbolic form of loving and repairing that arises from the logic of the depressive position.

From the depressive position, love is no longer pure, but burdened with guilt.[24] From that (so-called depressive) anxiety, the urge to recover is born. Many career choices, especially in healthcare and social work, reflect that desire for reparation. Something of the wounded inner object is sought in the patient, the student, or the client. The therapist repairs the mother, the nurse the brother, the teacher the lost child. However, Klein made it clear that repair is not quite the same as recovery. For example, the attempt at repair can actually reinforce the destruction if it stems from guilt. Goodwill can become coercion, empathy can become exhaustion. Sometimes, there is even a destructive component: aggressive impulses also find an outlet through career choices. In professions where power, control, or confrontation are central, the destructive drive is acted out and tamed. Klein thus shows that career choices always contain the tension between repair and destruction, between love and hate. The moral power of the reparative desire lies in the ability to tolerate ambivalence: love and hate, hope and guilt. The healthy therapist is not the unharmed one, but the one who has learned to symbolise their own aggression.

In more academic terms, Melanie Klein shifted the focus from instinct to object relations. According to her, every human being carries an inner world full of internalised images of parental figures—idealising or haunting, loving or vengeful. When these inner objects are damaged, the subject tries to repair them symbolically. From this perspective, career choice can be understood as a form of repair. The nurse or therapist heals in the other what once felt broken in their own psychological world. The inner ambivalence of human beings (the simultaneous desire to heal and to hurt) is transformed into an ethical framework within the profession. Psychoanalysis makes it clear that this ethic is not purely rational, but rooted in a deep inner need to repair what is broken inside. Nor is the dynamic described purely pathological. Yet there is also danger lurking in the reparative endeavour. After all, it can turn into excessive responsibility, perfectionism, or saviour behaviour.

Winnicott: Play and the Self

Donald Winnicott also separated sublimation from its instinctual roots and, in his own way, placed it within the relational. For him, the precursor to sublimation is not a defence against the drive but childlike play. This play unfolds in a potential or transitional space between mother and child. It is a space of illusion that arises from a good-enough mother who creates a holding environment. The transitional object (teddy bear, blanket, song) is the first building block of symbolisation and the first creative act. It is simultaneously discovered and invented in a kind of joint venture with the mother. It exists in an intermediate zone of experience that serves as the basis for all subsequent cultural and creative production. Winnicott explicitly distances himself from Freud in this regard:

> I am therefore introducing a new idea, that in the use of the object the infant destroys the object… The object survives destruction. This quality of 'surviving' is the key that unlocks the infant's use of the object… This change… means that the object is now a phenomenon in the external world, not a projective entity.[25]

Sublimation, and all the culture it implies, is a direct descendant of the ability to play in a transitional space where objects can be destroyed in fantasy but survive in reality. The painter's canvas, the composer's score, the writer's book, or the scientist's laboratory are all offshoots of the potential space. As in the cinema, they require both a suspension of belief and a suspension of disbelief.

On the one hand, the film being shown is more than just light passing through successive images; on the other hand, the bullets fired in it do not actually reach the audience. Sublimation is not a drive that is deflected, but a way of experiencing that dates back to our childhood and springs from a secure mother-child relationship. It revolves more around the (co)creation of a shared reality than around the discharge of personal energy.

Donald Winnicott subsequently introduced the distinction between the true and the false self in this line of thinking.[26] The true self is rooted in the spontaneous creativity and play described above, while the false self arises when the child must adapt to the needs of its environment at an early age. He also argued that children can only be themselves in an environment that tolerates their spontaneity. Otherwise, they fabricate a socially useful shell that protects the vulnerability of the true self. This echoes in many life stories: an identity that seeks to respond more to the demands of others than to inner feelings. Burnout, perfectionism, and chronic dissatisfaction are not signs of weakness in this constellation, but rather symptoms of a false self. Work, which was once supposed to be an expression of vitality, becomes a form of armour. For Winnicott, healing from this problem consists of (re)discovering the ability to play, to fail, and to breathe again. In this sense, choosing a career is a search for a place where play remains possible. He also emphasised that true vitality only arises when you feel connected to your spontaneous impulses.[27] The choice of career resonates with inner creativity and meaning, avoiding feelings of emptiness and exhaustion. Burnout, professional fatigue, or existential dissatisfaction can, on the other hand, be understood psychoanalytically as signs of alienation, as you allowed yourself to be 'trapped' by the needs of the Big Other.

Lacan: From Thing to Big Other

In his famous return to Freud, Jacques Lacan uses structuralism and linguistics to blend Freud's drive theory with a focus on the symbolic register. For him, the drive is inherently structured by language and the lack of being it causes. His most detailed discussion of sublimation appears in his seventh seminar, *The Ethics of Psychoanalysis* (1959–1960). There, he defines it succinctly as follows: 'Sublimation is the satisfaction of the drive without repression… it raises an object… to the dignity of the Thing (Das Ding).'[28] This Thing is Lacan's term for the lost and original object of desire: the unattainable maternal Thing from which we are permanently separated by a linguistic barrier. It is a hole or a void around which our desires gravitate. It is indeed like the sun: we cannot look at it or we will go blind, we cannot get too close or we will burn, but at too great a distance we suffer from a lack of warmth and light. For Lacan, sublimation is primarily about an object (a painting, a poem, a scientific idea) that covers and conceals the empty place of the Thing. This does not fulfil a (biological) need, but gives our desire a new symbolic form. Through artistic, scientific or religious creation, the libido is not channelled towards a new goal. Rather, the object is transfigured so that it makes the horror and/or awe of the Thing somewhat palpable. In this way, this object, promoted/sublimated to the Thing, provides a profound and paradoxical form of satisfaction. After all, in Lacan's view, the drive cannot reach the object. Instead, it circles around it symbolically and imaginarily.

Jacques Lacan also radicalised Freud's insights, arguing that the subject's desire is always mediated by the Big Other. We do not desire spontaneously, but in relation to the symbolic signifiers that the Other presents us with. Human desire is the desire of the Other: we want what the Other wants or wants us to want. Career choice is therefore not an autonomous decision, but an answer to the implicit question: what does the Other want me to become? Parents, culture, and society prescribe signifiers: doctor, engineer, teacher, actor, nurse, psychologist. Each profession embodies a position within the symbolic order, namely, a place where the subject hopes to find recognition.

The object petit a is, as it were, the echo of the Thing in the realm of the senses. It is also the object that causes desire. It plays just as crucial a role as the vanishing point in a painting. It is invisible yet constitutive of every representation. In every profession, we seek what is missing: admiration, recognition, love, power, or meaning. But because the *object a* is by definition unattainable, the choice of profession retains the structure of an endless quest. In Lacan's theory, the phallus in turn functions as a signifier of desire and law. It is that which we can never have or be enough to (completely) satisfy the desire of the Big Other. Many career choices have a phallic dimension: status, prestige, and power mask the underlying lack. In this way, the profession becomes not only a form of economic activity but also a symbol of success: an attempt to ward off the lack. The phallic logic (I am or I have 'it' for the Other) structures many professional ambitions. The professional who believes he is 'Someone' thereby covers up the emptiness that drives him. The analyst distinguishes himself only by being (more fully) aware that his practice also revolves precisely around that emptiness.

Calling, Vocation, and Profession

After this psychoanalytical *tour d'horizon* of career choices in general, I will now take a closer look at calling, vocation, and profession.[29] In their intertwined nature, they play an important role in the choice of care professions. These are three concepts that overlap but still have (slightly) different meanings. Our private desires can be connected to the Big Other in various ways and to varying degrees.

In religious and cultural traditions, a calling suggests an external summons—a voice or command from beyond the self—that demands recognition. A vocation implies a more inwardly appropriated sense of destiny or purpose, an identity shaped through unconscious identifications and expectations. A profession refers to the institutional and symbolic inscription of this trajectory within a social framework governed by rules, ethics, and collective standards. Psychoanalysis offers a privileged perspective to disentangle these registers, for it is attentive to the unconscious forces that motivate occupational choices, the transference of love and authority into professional life, and the sublimatory potential that transforms drives into socially recognised activities.

Calling

A calling, in its etymological roots, designates the *voice* that summons. In classical Christian traditions, the idea of 'the call' referred to divine vocation, the sense that one's life path is chosen not by the individual but by God. Psychoanalysis reframes this in terms of the unconscious Big Other: the injunction of the Superego, the parental voice internalised, the interpellation of the subject by a desire (or demand) that is not their own. Freud's reflections on occupational choice already hinted at this dimension. He observed that many analysts were drawn to the profession not merely by intellectual curiosity but by an unconscious need to repair personal wounds.[30] He noted the 'motives of suffering and of healing' that recur in those who feel summoned to psychoanalysis. This resonates with what can be named a *calling*: a compulsion to answer to a voice that speaks from the site of one's own symptom. For Freud, the voice of the superego represents the harshest form of this calling, the demand to be worthy in the eyes of an internalised parental figure.[31]

Lacan radicalised this view by situating the voice as one of the manifestations of object a. In his tenth seminar on anxiety, Lacan identified the voice as a partial object that operates beyond the realm of meaning.[32] A calling, then, can be heard as the subject's encounter with the enigmatic voice of the Other, which interrupts existence with an imperative that may never be fully understood. To feel 'called' is to be seized by a lack in being. It is what Lacan described as the *manque-à-être* or want-to-be. The individual perceives that their life is not their own but is oriented by an enigmatic desire that requires a response.

Christopher Bollas introduced the notion of the 'destiny drive,' a psychic tendency that impels individuals toward experiences and pursuits that actualise deeply buried aspects of their idiom.[33] What appears as a calling is, in this sense, the expression of a deep organisation of unconscious life that seeks recognition in the external world. Bollas emphasises that such callings are not purely determined by external command but resonate with the 'unthought known' of the subject's early life. Thus, calling can be understood psychoanalytically as the moment when the unconscious speaks through the guise of destiny. It represents an encounter with alterity (whether divine, parental, or that of the Superego) that insists upon a path of life. Yet, because the voice of the Other is never transparent, the subject risks mistaking coercion for inspiration, guilt for purpose, and symptom for mission.

Vocation

While calling stresses the voice from beyond, vocation concerns the way individuals internalise this voice as their own destiny. The Latin *vocare* (to call) persists, but here it signals not only an external summons but an inward alignment: a life path that feels fatefully *meant to be*. Psychoanalytically, vocation highlights the role of identification, parentification, and the unconscious transmission of desire.

Freud, in his case study of *Little Hans*, noted that children's fantasies of occupation are linked to Oedipal identifications: boys imagine becoming like their fathers, girls like their mothers, to secure love and recognition.[34] Vocation is therefore tied to unconscious familial dramas. Choosing a life path may be less about authentic self-discovery than about fulfilling the parental unconscious. When a child 'takes up the vocation' of becoming a doctor, solicitor, or artist, it is often a way of inhabiting the wish of the Other.

Jessica Benjamin highlighted how vocation often involves the paradox of recognition.[35] To follow a vocation is to seek to be recognised by those who matter, yet at the same time to assert one's own recognition of oneself as agent. This creates an ambivalence: the vocation is never purely one's own but entangled with the desire to satisfy or repair the objects of one's love. In psychoanalytic training, for example, many candidates discover that their vocation is bound to the desire to heal parents or repeat childhood scenes of caretaking.

From the perspective of object relations theory, vocation functions as a *reparative project*. Melanie Klein already suggested that sublimation is often motivated by the wish to restore damaged internal objects.[36] A vocation in teaching, medicine, or psychoanalysis may thus emerge as an unconscious effort to repair a beloved but wounded maternal imago. Vocation is not simply the pursuit of talent; it is a dialogue with internal object worlds.

Adam Phillips has noted that vocation often masks compulsion.[37] The story of 'finding one's vocation' is narrated retroactively as destiny, but beneath it lies an economy of unconscious repetition. The individual may proclaim, 'I was born to be a therapist,' when in fact their vocation expresses an unresolved identification with a depressive or dependent parent. Phillips cautions that vocation can become a trap: an idealisation that conceals the impossibility of ever truly fulfilling the Big Other's demand.

Thus, vocation psychoanalytically represents the *subjective appropriation* of a calling. It is how the subject translates the voice of the Other into the language of destiny, turning unconscious injunctions into a personal narrative of purpose. But vocation remains haunted by ambivalence: it can liberate through sublimation or enslave through compulsive repetition.

Profession

A profession, finally and by contrast, introduces a symbolic dimension. It is no longer the intimate drama of unconscious desire but the inscription of one's work within the structures of society. A profession is defined by institutions, diplomas, ethical codes, and collective recognition. It situates the subject not only in relation to parents or unconscious voices, but also to the law, tradition, and peers.

Freud himself was attentive to the dangers of unregulated vocations. In his debates about lay analysis, he insisted on the importance of training, supervision, and institutional frameworks. While he opened psychoanalysis to non-medical practitioners, Freud underlined that without professional regulation, the practice risked collapsing into personal enthusiasm or charismatic authority.[38] The profession, then, provides a symbolic boundary that protects both patient and practitioner from the excesses of private compulsion.

Lacan emphasised the role of the *Name-of-the-Father* as the signifier that anchors the subject in the symbolic order.[39] A profession can be seen as one such paternal function: it grants a title, a place, and a recognition that regulates desire. The analyst, for instance, does not practise as a private vocation alone but as inscribed within a school, an institution, a symbolic community. The profession guards against psychotic foreclosure by ensuring that the subject's work is recognised within the symbolic order.

Profession also implies the management of narcissism. Kernberg argued that professional identity integrates both narcissistic investments (pride, status) and sublimatory aims (serving society).[40] A healthy professional stance requires balancing these elements, preventing omnipotent fantasies of healing while sustaining motivation. Professional ethics, licensure, and peer review provide external support for this internal balance. The profession is therefore the site where unconscious vocation is translated into symbolic law. It demands a submission of private destiny to collective standards. It also introduces a tension: the professional role may constrain the authenticity of one's vocation, but without it the vocation risks turning into obsession or delusion.

Interplay

The three registers are best seen as dynamically interrelated. A calling confronts us with the enigmatic voice of the Other, a vocation appropriates this voice into the narrative of self, a profession inscribes this narrative into the symbolic order. Each contains risks, such as fanaticism, compulsive repetition, and bureaucratic alienation, but also holds potential for meaning, creativity, and love. In clinical terms, analysts often hear patients struggle with these registers. Some experience their work as a calling, perhaps compelled to care for others at the expense of their own well-being. Others narrate their vocation as a family drama: 'I became a doctor because my father never could.' Still others struggle with the constraints of the profession, including burnout resulting from institutional demands, ethical conflicts, or the erosion of passion under bureaucratic pressures. The analytic task is to help subjects disentangle these threads, recognising where desire ends and coercion begins. Psychoanalysis teaches us that no life path is purely rational or autonomous. What appears as destiny is often repetition; what feels like freedom may conceal compulsion. Yet, within the dialectic of calling, vocation, and profession lies the possibility of sublimation: the transformation of private wounds into socially meaningful work.

Psychoanalytic Motives

I return to some psychoanalytic motives for psychological counsellors that have been neglected so far. In addition to the life instinct (Eros), Freud also introduced the death instinct (Thanatos).[41] On the one hand, there is the desire to connect, heal, and create; on the other hand, there is the fascination with destruction, aggression, and death. Therapists are inevitably confronted with the death drive in the destructive impulses of their patients, but also in their own inner world. The helping profession can be seen as an attempt to tame these destructive forces, to symbolise them, and to bring them into a workable dialogue with Eros. This dialectic gives the profession its psychological intensity and existential weight.

Parallel to this, of course, is the distinction between libido and aggression. Libido is focused on connecting with the other, while aggression is about distancing oneself from the other and autonomy.[42] The profession of psychotherapist can function as a reaction formation against feelings of sadism, hatred, and aggression.[43] Through their profession, therapists aim to demonstrate that they are not destructive or harmful.[44] A controlled expression of feelings of hatred is, especially in very serious cases, useful and possibly even necessary.[45] I refer to Winnicott's famous article on hatred in countertransference.[46] In this context, masochism refers conversely to an (unconscious) attraction to pain and suffering in the individual.[47] I quote Michael Sussman:

> There appears to be a masochistic element to the very desire to expose oneself to those who are ill and disturbed. ... There must be a certain degree of masochism in the therapist to accept the patient's hostility and other strong feelings without reciprocating.[48]

The literature also frequently refers to narcissistic motives in working as a therapist. Again, Sussman writes: 'The role of psychotherapist may be viewed as an attempt to overcome the narcissistic damage of having been inappropriately "used" by a parent at a point in development where the roles should have been reversed.'[49]

Therapists who shy away from feelings of dependence may also be able to meet this need through their work. By caring for the other person and identifying with them, the need for dependence is indirectly fulfilled. The underlying desire is usually to provide the other person with something that the therapist themselves missed out on—for example, their parents or their own therapist. According to Sussman, many therapists have a strong need for intimacy on the one hand, but on the other hand, they also have fears surrounding this same theme.[50]

Finally, the epistemophilic drive (*Ger.: Wisstrieb*) also plays a crucial role. Freud regarded this as a fundamental desire for knowledge and understanding.[51] Christopher Bollas, for example, introduced the category of the 'unthought known': aspects of psychological experience that are present but not symbolically expressed.[52] The psychotherapist is driven by the desire to bring this unthought into language and relationship. For her part, Jessica Benjamin emphasised the relational dimension: therapists seek not only knowledge, but also a dialectical recognition of the self in the other.[53] For them, psychotherapy is a search for meaning, reciprocity, and a place in an intersubjective field. The choice of a therapeutic profession is therefore also an answer to existential questions: how can one live with rupture, division, and desire?

The Wounded Healer

It should be clear by now. The conscious motivation to help people is socially desirable and professionally accepted, but the therapist's career choice is often driven by unconscious, complex motives.[54] What we consciously think we know about ourselves is only part of the story; a sceptical attitude towards our conscious intentions is advisable.[55] Within a large part of the profession, there appear to be significant emotional issues as a result of early childhood experiences.[56] The desire to assist others may be a veiled way of remedying something within ourselves or compensating for past shortcomings. Glen Gabbard emphasises that, in line with this, in addition to altruistic intentions, there is usually also a more unconscious desire to free ourselves from inner difficulties, as well as a striving to satisfy previously unfulfilled needs.[57] Elvin Semrad, an American psychiatrist, is said to have described psychotherapy as 'an encounter between a mess and an even bigger mess.'[58]

My compatriot Myriam Van Gael even sees the therapist almost *by definition* as a 'wounded healer.'[59] Research indeed shows that therapists do not really come from average families.[60] Psychology and psychiatry students report greater emotional stress in their early childhood than students in other fields. Research suggests that psychotherapists are more likely than other professional groups to come from problematic families, with a higher risk of affective disorders, alcoholism, or psychiatric problems among their parents.[61] Childhood traumas such as physical or sexual abuse and experiences of loss are also above average.[62] The career choice of psychotherapists is often complex and multi-layered. In addition to altruism, intellectual challenge, autonomy, and the search for self-understanding also play a role.[63] Many hope to get to know themselves better or to heal through their work.[64] Others experience the therapeutic role as a safe form of intimacy that circumvents their fear of closeness.[65] According to Adam Phillips, for Winnicott, caring for his depressed mother was a lifelong motivation to help others.[66]

Narcissistic wounds also play a role. Therapists may seek power and control in the dependent relationship with clients, which confirms their self-image but can also lead to boundary violations. The concept of the 'wounded healer' emphasises how personal pain can motivate powerful help-giving, but it can just as easily lead to problematic identifications and projections.[67]

A disproportionate number of therapists come from families with significant psychopathology (depression, schizophrenia, severe personality disorders, and alcoholism) and/or have experienced traumatic events such as deprivation of parental care, personal illness, death of a parent, or divorce. They were often the oldest or parentified child, and their vocation is the symptomatic result of inner conflicts.[68] These inner conflicts can revolve around aggression and feelings of guilt. Dedicated therapists can appease their conscience by transcending anger, hatred, and envy thanks to the nature of their work.[69] They may have issues with connection and intimacy that can be satisfied and resolved through their work within a psychotherapeutic framework. However, no motivation for the care provider is mentioned as often as that related to narcissistic gratification such as the need for power or omnipotence.[70] Thanks to transference, does the therapist not often become a beloved and adored God in the depths of the patient's mind?

In her bestseller *The Drama of the Gifted Child*, Alice Miller convincingly demonstrated the link between narcissistic problems and a career in social work.[71] Adults who were parentified as children can become therapists who always want to feel important and go the extra mile. They are constantly searching for the recognition they never received. They work themselves to the bone in self-sacrificing responsibility and justice, but instead of confirmation, they often reap annoyance or envy because of the pioneering role they repeatedly take on, driven but unsolicited. Indeed, the profession of therapist is, in Sussman's ambiguous formulation, *A Curious Calling*.[72] A curious calling because it is motivated by curiosity, for example about (bedroom and other) secrets. But also a curious calling because it has a certain (morbid, perverse, or sinful) odour attached to it. If, and only if, the care provider is sufficiently 'cured' of such 'unhealthy' curiosity, can he combine professional and experiential expertise. Memories and desires[73] are not absent from him, but they are sufficiently purified to be suspended for the benefit of the patient. The therapist normally receives a wage and sometimes even an honorarium for his work. This is very different from the parentified child who, in any case (as a child), felt abandoned and/or used. In a sense, they get a slap in the face for their efforts because they are curtailed and crippled in their own development in all kinds of ways. Their wages are paid, so to speak, in Monopoly money. At best, their validity is limited to the domestic sphere.

Psychological Counselling

The step from choosing a profession in general to choosing psychological counselling in particular thus reveals specific psychodynamics. Care providers and therapists are often driven by a desire to heal, understand, or bring meaning, but this motivation is rarely purely altruistic. Behind the desire to help often lies a personal history of hurt. This motive is classically expressed in the image of the *wounded healer*. The archetype of the wounded healer goes back to the Greek figure of Chiron. This immortal centaur was struck by a poisonous arrow and remained wounded forever. His suffering did not prevent him from healing others; on the contrary, it became the source of his wisdom. This myth depicts the paradox that healing comes from one's own vulnerability. Carl Gustav Jung popularised this image.[74] According to him, every doctor or therapist is both a healer and a wounded person: 'A doctor is effective only in so far as he has met his own wounded self.' It is precisely the confrontation with one's own suffering that forms the basis for empathy and healing. Zerubavel and Wright elaborate on this archetype.[75] They show that the therapist's 'backpack' has a dual function: it can be a source of strength, but also a risk. It is a strength because those who have experienced suffering themselves have an increased capacity for empathy and tolerance: the therapist can *endure* the pain of others because they know their own pain. They know psychological problems inside and out. Certainly, after undergoing their own analysis, little that is human (and even inhuman) is foreign to them. But at the same time, there is also a risk. If their own wounds have not been sufficiently processed, there is a danger of over-identification. The therapist may unconsciously use the patient to heal their own scars. They emphasise that 'being wounded' only becomes healing when it is symbolically processed. Supervision, self-reflection, and personal therapy are therefore not a luxury, but a structural requirement.

Freud himself warned of the analyst's inevitable blind spots: unprocessed conflicts in the analyst's unconscious can disrupt the transference.[76] Both he and Sàndor Ferenczi emphasised that personal psychoanalysis is a must in order to prevent this as much as possible.[77] Ferenczi also emphasised authenticity and affective resonance: the therapist must acknowledge their own vulnerability without projecting it onto the patient.[78] From a Kleinian perspective, projective identification plays a crucial role. The patient may unconsciously exploit the therapist's unresolved wounds. He recruits the therapist to download certain content into him like a kind of virus program, and when the therapist does not recognise or acknowledge this, he begins to feel and behave accordingly. Only those who have symbolised their own pain can transform such projections into meaning.

Winnicott spoke about the *holding environment*: the therapist can only offer a safe space if he himself is sufficiently 'held.'[79] An unhealed wound leads to an unstable *holding:* the therapist uses the patient to hold himself. Bion described the therapist as *a container* for the patient's raw contents/beta elements.[80] The wounded healer is extra sensitive to these emotional storms; he can understand them better but is also more likely to be overwhelmed by them. The therapist is a vessel for the patient's projections; he must not repel them but tolerate them. Yet the container itself can burst when the contents exceed its capacity. Finally, Lacan reminds us that every analyst carries his own symptom. The question is not whether he is wounded, but whether he can structure his wound in such a way that it becomes a condition for action rather than an obstacle. In doing so, the analyst works not against but with his symptom.

Empirical studies confirm this tension and its ambiguous nature. Rek et al. found that psychotherapy trainees score lower on avoidant attachment and higher on harmonious interpersonal motives than control groups: they long for closeness and feel comfortable in intimate relationships.[81] Fussell and Bonney showed that therapists reported significantly more trauma or emotional deprivation in their childhood, which deepened their interest and increased their sensitivity.[82] Lester Luborsky showed that *the therapist's personality* is a determining factor in treatment success, often more so than the method used.[83] These data suggest that personal wounds and interpersonal sensitivity are structurally related to the choice of and effectiveness in the helping profession.

Parentification as a Source and a Pitfall

Every calling to help starts somewhere. Sometimes in admiration, sometimes in need. Often, in that quiet moment, when a child notices that the parent is missing something (strength, joy, protection) the child decides to fill the void. What at first glance seems like simple love is also a form of self-denial. The line between giving oneself and disappearing becomes blurred. We saw, for example, that Gregory Jurkovic distinguished between functional and destructive parentification.[84] A little responsibility can grow into caring and maturity; chronic responsibility, however, can undermine childlike vitality. Those who have to care too early also do not learn enough about what it means to receive. Lisa Hooper described how parentification leads to a paradox: the child develops empathy as a survival strategy, but later carries that empathy as a burden.[85] John Bowlby described this as *compulsive caregiving*: providing care to avoid one's own dependence.[86] As adults, they exhibit an attachment style in which giving is central, but receiving remains difficult.[87] The parentified adult often becomes a therapist, doctor, educator, or teacher: someone who once again absorbs the pain of others because they were never allowed to show their own. In that light, the choice to provide psychological help is not purely altruistic, but existential: an attempt to heal in others what remained unspoken in themselves.

A particularly striking example of the *wounded healer* is indeed the parentified therapist. Hidden within them is a child who became the confidant, comforter, or carer of their parent. Jurkovic emphasised that it is not the act itself that is harmful, but its chronic and unequal nature.[88] Parentification always has ambivalent effects.[89] On the one hand, it promotes empathy, responsibility, and sensitivity: qualities that are very useful later on in social work. On the other hand, it can lead to feelings of guilt, role confusion, depression, and burnout. The parentified therapist, therefore, embodies a paradox: his early-acquired caring identity makes him exceptionally sensitive to the needs of others, but at the same time vulnerable to excessive involvement.

From a psychoanalytical point of view, the parentified therapist is prey to repetition compulsion. We have discussed what Freud would say: the parentified therapist repeats what he cannot remember. The childish fantasy of saving the parent is revived in relation to the suffering patient. The unconscious urge to care and be recognised can undermine neutrality. Ferenczi would speak of a confusion of tongues.[90] The therapist still speaks the language of the child who bore responsibility for the adult world. Childish and adult registers thus become mixed up and confused. The parentified therapist risks repeating the same confusion in treatment: he identifies too strongly with the needy child in the patient. When sufficiently placed and understood, this resonance opens the possibility of deeper authenticity. Unbearable affects are disowned and, as it were, downloaded into the other person. Unnoticed, the virus program unfolds in this recipient. A parentified therapist, accustomed to carrying others' feelings, is particularly receptive to such projections. If symbolisation is lacking, collusion arises; if present, exceptional insight arises. Melanie Klein saw this attitude as a variant of repair.[91] Winnicott would add that the parentified counsellor knows how to *hold*, but not how *to be held*. He offers security but does not know it from within. Bion would describe it as an overly porous *container*: it tolerates everything until it evaporates. And Lacan would argue that the parentified therapist chooses his profession in response to the desire or need of the Other in an attempt to embody *object a* that the Other once lacked. The symptom of the parentified psychotherapist is compulsive caring for the other. This symptom does not so much need to be erased as it needs to serve the process, not the repetition. Lacan's idea also applies here: enjoy your symptom![92]

In clinical practice, we recognise recurring problems. Parentified psychotherapists tend to display an excessive sense of responsibility, which makes it difficult for them to let patients struggle and fail. The boundaries can be somewhat vague, leading to a tendency to overcommit or to be available outside of sessions. Rescuer fantasies can result in countertransference focusing more on caring and protecting than on interpreting. Narcissistic motives can lead to abuse of the patient's dependence. Winnicott emphasised that it is precisely the capacity to tolerate failure that is essential: the therapist must learn to live with imperfection and the realisation that not everything can be repaired.[93] Parentified therapists are also more vulnerable to exhaustion and burnout, repeating earlier self-sacrifice and suffering under the burden of care or even succumbing to it. For patients, these idiosyncrasies of their psychotherapist can be both healing and risky. They often feel intensely seen, but the relationship can become symbiotic. The therapist must therefore constantly balance empathy and distance. The child who once carried too much now carries too much as a therapist. The path to sufficient professionalism is to transform the wound into an instrument.

Conclusion

All this requires, first and foremost, sufficient personal analysis to clarify the distinction between past parentification and current professional responsibility. Nancy McWilliams also warns that the profession requires constant self-reflection and self-analysis to avoid pitfalls.[94] Psychotherapists in training have a similar 'baggage' in terms of adverse childhood events as the wider population. However, a high percentage of them have been able to build a secure attachment and their mentalising ability is also above average. Both the quality of their attachment and the number of hours of personal therapy temper the effect of early childhood negative experiences on their reflective functioning.[95]

Supervision is also important in order to recognise enactments and rescue dynamics in a timely and sufficient manner. Adequate self-care and boundaries are points of attention to prevent the old self-sacrifice from being repeated. For Van Gael, self-care is not merely self-interest, but an ethical duty.[96] After all, the effectiveness of therapy depends heavily on the therapist as a person. The American Psychological Association's Code of Ethics explicitly states that psychologists must be aware of the influence of their own health on their work and, if necessary, limit their activities or seek help.[97] Self-care naturally requires awareness first and foremost: therapists must learn to recognise their own risk factors and warning signs. Examples include irritability towards clients, hoping that appointments will be cancelled, or compensatory behaviour such as alcohol consumption.[98]

Specific terms describe the psychological burden on therapists. Therapist distress refers to signs of exhaustion, insomnia, and emotional withdrawal, often associated with prolonged stress.[99] Therapist impairment occurs when this distress remains untreated and affects functioning: clinical judgement weakens, boundaries become blurred, and the risk of deontological and ethical errors increases.[100] Subtypes include compassion fatigue, burnout, and secondary traumatisation.[101] Risk factors include a high caseload, many traumatised patients, and isolation from colleagues. The impact of the work extends into the private sphere. Many therapists experience emotional exhaustion after work, making them less receptive to the daily concerns of their partner and children.[102] This often leads to relationship tensions, divorce, or a feeling of isolation.[103]

An important counterbalance to distress lies in continuous professional development. Orlinsky and Rønnestad conducted an international study of more than 12,000 therapists.[104] They identified two dimensions: healing involvement (connectedness, flow, effectiveness) and stressful involvement (difficulties, avoidance coping, anxiety). What promotes healing involvement is primarily the experience of growth: the feeling of developing and learning from daily practice. Supervision and further training contribute to this, but therapists learn most from their clients themselves. This experience of growth has a remoralising effect and protects against burnout.

In order not to deny the history of parentification, but to integrate it as a source of empathy, sufficient symbolisation and mentalisation are necessary in any case. As Bion stated, it is not a matter of avoiding projections, but of transforming them into *thinkable thoughts*.[105] When the therapist can reflect on their history rather than repeat it, the wound becomes an effective factor in the transference. By symbolising the history of parentification, the wound is not erased but tamed. It must be thought about, not repeated. Only then does the unfinished become the finished past and fate become story and history.

Thinking is the ennoblement of suffering, and the wound is a path. Psychoanalysis teaches us that the wound does not disappear, but changes location. It shifts from scar to symbol. The counsellor who knows his history no longer needs to restore what has been lost. He can listen. And in that listening, the wound becomes something else: a place where the other person can speak without judgment. I therefore conclude the psychoanalysis of our career choice not diagnostically but (with permission) poetically. It always says the same thing: your choice is a sentence, written with the alphabet of your past. And therapy is the reading of that sentence, until it takes on meaning instead of imposing its compulsion on you.

Notes

1 As the psychiatrist responsible for treatment policy in a clinical psychotherapeutic programme in a psychiatric institution, see Kinet (2024).
2 De Cauter (2011, p. 193 ff.).
3 Bregman (2024, p. 69).
4 Sussman (1992).
5 Staal (2024) also refers to Malach-Pines and Yafe-Yenai (1999).
6 Freud (1914).
7 Freud (1920a).
8 Levy et al. (2006).
9 Solms (2021); Kinet (2023).
10 Gabbard (2014).
11 de Gaulejac (1987. p. 13). My transl: man is the product of a history of which he tries to become the subject.
12 Laplanche and Pontalis (1973 p. 432).
13 In Masson (1985, p. 287).
14 Freud (1905).
15 Freud (1905, p. 178).
16 Freud (1910, p. 223).
17 Freud (1930, p. 97).
18 Freud (1908).
19 Freud (1937a).
20 Freud (1921).
21 Freud (1937b).
22 Duchamp (1957, p. 139).
23 Klein (1957, p. 210).
24 Klein (1935).
25 Winnicott (1971, p. 48).
26 Winnicott (1960).
27 Winnicott (1965).
28 Lacan (1959–1960, p. 133).
29 Duffy and Dik (2013); Wrzesniewski et al. (1997).
30 Freud (1926),
31 Freud (1923).
32 Lacan (1962–1963).
33 Bollas (1992).
34 Freud (1909).
35 Benjamin (1995).
36 Klein (1935).
37 Phillips (1993).
38 Freud (1926).

39 Lacan (1957–1958).
40 Kernberg (1975).
41 Freud (1920).
42 De Wolf (2015).
43 Gabbard and Wilkinson (2000).
44 Maroda (2022).
45 Gabbard and Wilkinson (2000).
46 Winnicott (1958).
47 Lingiardi and McWilliams (2018).
48 Sussman (1992, p. 84).
49 Sussman (1992, p. 125).
50 Sussman (1992, p. 125).
51 'A strong impulse of curiosity arises in the child, directed to the problem of sexual life. This impulse cannot be regarded as a derivative of the sexual instinct; rather, it is to be classed as a component instinct in its own right: the instinct for knowledge [*Wiss-trieb*]' (Freud, 1905, p. 194). We now know for certain that we simply share the emotional-instinctive SEEKING system with mammals (Panksepp, 1998).
52 Bollas (1987).
53 Benjamin (1990).
54 Norcross and Farber (2005).
55 Lemma (2015).
56 Barnett et al. (2007).
57 Gabbard (2000).
58 Mintz (2015, p.190).
59 Van Gael (2000 pp. 4, 10).
60 Van Gael (1998).
61 Farber et al. (2005).
62 Dickeson, Mazerolle, and Pitney (2017).
63 Murphy and Halgin (1995); Norcross and Farber (2005).
64 Barnett et al. (2007).
65 Farber et al. (2005).
66 Phillips (2007).
67 Cain (2000); Conchar and Repper (2014).
68 Winer (1994).
69 Gabbard (1995).
70 Donnay-Richelle , Timsit, and Dongier (1972), Finell (1985), Van Gael (2000, p. 8; 2020).
71 Miller (1979).
72 Sussman (1992).
73 Bion (1970).
74 Jung (1951, p. 69).
75 Zerubavel and Wright (2012).
76 Freud (1912).
77 'Anyone who wishes to practise analysis on others should first be analysed himself' (Freud 1912, p. 115) or 'A doctor's own analysis is the best school for learning the practice of analysis' (Freud 1926, p. 246). See also 'The analyst must be analysed as deeply as possible; otherwise he will infect his patient with his own complexes' (Ferenczi 1928, p. 93).
78 Ferenczi (1932).
79 Winnicott (1965).
80 Bion (1962).
81 Rek et al. (2018).

82 Fussell and Bonney (1990).
83 Luborsky et al. (1986).
84 Jurkovic (1997).
85 Hooper (2008).
86 Bowlby (1977).
87 West and Keller (1991).
88 Jurkovic (1997).
89 Hooper (2008); Masiran et al. (2023).
90 Ferenczi (1932).
91 Klein (1946).
92 Žižek (1992).
93 Winnicott (1965).
94 McWilliams (2004).
95 Klasen et al. (2019).
96 Van Gael (2020).
97 Barnett et al. (2007).
98 Norcross and VandenBos (2018).
99 Barnett et al. (2007).
100 Smith and Moss (2009).
101 Laverdière et al. (2019).
102 Råbu et al. (2016).
103 Kennedy and Black (2010).
104 Orlinsky and Rønnestad (2005).
105 Bion (1962).

References

Barnett, J. E., Baker, E. K., Elman, N. S., and Schoener, G. R. (2007). In pursuit of wellness: The self-care imperative. *Professional Psychology: Research and Practice*, 38, 603–612.

Benjamin, J. (1990). *The Bonds of Love: Psychoanalysis, Feminism, and the Problem of Domination*. New York: Pantheon Books.

Benjamin, J. (1995). *Like Subjects, Love Objects: Essays on Recognition and Sexual Difference*. New Haven, CT: Yale University Press.

Bion, W. R. (1962). *Learning from Experience*. London: Heinemann.

Bion, W. R. (1970). *Attention and Interpretation*. London: Karnac.

Bollas, C. (1987). *The Shadow of the Object: Psychoanalysis of the Unthought Known*. London: Free Association Books.

Bollas, C. (1992). *Being a Character: Psychoanalysis and Self Experience*. New York: Hill and Wang.

Bowlby, J. (1977). The making and breaking of affectional bonds: II. Some principles of psychotherapy: The Fiftieth Maudsley Lecture (expanded version). *The British Journal of Psychiatry*, 130(5), 421–431. doi:10.1192/bjp.130.5.421

Bregman, R. (2024). *Moral Ambition: Stop Wasting Your Talent and Start Making a Difference*. New York: Bloomsbury.

Cain, N. R. (2000). Psychotherapists with personal histories of psychiatric hospitalization. *Psychiatric Rehabilitation Journal*, 24, 22–28. https://psycnet.apa.org/doi/10.1037/h0095127

Conchar, C., and Repper, J. (2014). 'Walking wounded or wounded healer?' Does personal experience of mental health problems help or hinder mental health practice? A review of the literature. *Mental Health and Social Inclusion*, 18, 35–44. doi:10.1108/MHSI-02-2014-0003

De Cauter, L (2011). *De Oorsprongen of het Boek der Verbazing*. Leuven: LannooCampus.

de Gaulejac, V. (1987). *La névrose de classe: trajectoire sociale et conflits d'identité*. Paris: Hommes et Groupes éditeurs.

De Wolf, M. H. M. (2015). *Psychoanalytische theorievorming en de DSM-5*. Bussum: Coutinho.

Dickeson, E., Mazerolle, S. M., and Pitney, W. A. (2017). The prevalence and implications of wounded healers: A systematic review of the literature. *Athletic Training Education Journal*, 12(4), 276–286. doi:10.4085/1204276

Donnay-Richelle, J., Timsit, M. and Dongier, M. (1972). Study of the deep motivations of vocational choice in psychiatry candidates and students in psychology. *Acta Psychiatrica Belgica*, 72, 345–346.

Duchamp, M. (1957). The creative act. In: A. Sanouillet and E. Peterson (eds), *The Writings of Marcel Duchamp*. New York: Da Capo Press, 1973.

Duffy, R. D., and Dik, B. J. (2013). *Make Your Job a Calling: How the Psychology of Vocation Can Change Your Life at Work*. West Conshohocken: Templeton Press.

Farber, B. A., Manevich, I., Metzger, J., and Saypol, E. (2005). Choosing psychotherapy as a career: Why did we cross that road? *Journal of Clinical Psychology*, 61, 1009–1031. doi:10.1002/jclp.20174

Ferenczi, S. (1928). The elasticity of psycho-analytic technique. In M. Balint (ed.), *Final Contributions to the Problems and Methods of Psycho-Analysis* (pp. 87–101). London: Hogarth, 1955.

Ferenczi, S. (1932). *The Clinical Diary of Sándor Ferenczi* (M. Balint, ed.; M. Dupont, trans.). Cambridge, MA: Harvard University Press, 1988.

Finell, J. S. (1985). Narcissistic problems in analysts. *International Journal of Psychoanalytic Psychotherapy*, 9, 227–231.

Freud, S. (1905). Three essays on the theory of sexuality. In J. Strachey (ed. and trans.), *S. E.* (Vol. 7, pp. 125–245). London: Hogarth, 1953.

Freud, S. (1908). Character and anal erotism. In *S. E.* (Vol. 9, pp. 167–175). London: Hogarth.

Freud, S. (1910). 'Wild' psycho-analysis. In *S. E.* (Vol. 11, pp. 219–227). London: Hogarth, 1957.

Freud, S. (1912). Recommendations to physicians practising psycho-analysis. In *S. E.* (Vol. 12, pp. 109–120). London: Hogarth, 1958.

Freud, S. (1914). Remembering, repeating and working-through. In *S. E.* (Vol. 12, pp. 145–156). London: Hogarth, 1958.

Freud, S. (1920a). Aan gene zijde van het lustprincipe. In *Psychoanalytische theorie* (Vol. 1). Amsterdam: Boom.

Freud, S. (1920b). Beyond the pleasure principle. In *S. E.* (Vol. 18, pp. 1–64). London: Hogarth, 1961.

Freud, S. (1921). Group psychology and the analysis of the ego. In *S. E.* (Vol. 18, pp. 65–143). London: Hogarth, 1955.

Freud, S. (1923). The ego and the id. In *S. E.* (Vol. 19, pp. 12–66). London: Hogarth, 1961.

Freud, S. (1926). The question of lay analysis. In *S. E.* (Vol. 20, pp. 179–258). London: Hogarth, 1969.

Freud, S. (1930). Civilization and its discontents. In *S. E.* (Vol. 21, pp. 57–145). London: Hogarth, 1961.

Freud, S. (1937a). Analysis terminable and interminable. In *S. E.* (Vol. 23, pp. 209–254). London: Hogarth, 1964.

Freud, S. (1937b). Constructions in analysis. In *S. E.* (Vol. 23, pp. 255–270). London: Hogarth, 1964.

Fussell, F. W., and Bonney, W. C. (1990). A comparative study of childhood experiences of psychotherapists and physicists: Implications for clinical practice. *Psychotherapy: Theory, Research, Practice, Training*, 27 (4), 505–512.

Gabbard, G. O. (1995). When the patient is a therapist. Special challenges in the psychoanalysis of mental health professionals. *Psychoanalytic Review*, 82 pp. 709–725.

Gabbard, G. O. (2000). On gratitude and gratification. *Journal of the American Psychoanalytic Association*, 48 (3), 698–716.

Gabbard, G. O., and Wilkinson, S. M. (2000). *Management of Countertransference with Borderline Patients.* Plymouth, UK: Rowman and Littlefield Publishers, Inc.

Gabbard, G. O. (2014). *Psychodynamic Psychiatry in Clinical Practice* (5th edn). Washington, DC: American Psychiatric Publishing.

Hooper, L. M. (2008). Defining and understanding Parentification. *The Alabama Counseling Association Journal*, 34 (1), 34–43.

Jung, C. G. (1951). *Memories, Dreams, Reflections* (A. Jaffé, ed.; R. Winston and C. Winston, trans.). New York: Vintage, 1983.

Jurkovic, G. J. (1997). *Lost Childhoods: The Plight of the Parentified Child.* New York: Brunner/Mazel, 2014.

Kennedy, B. S., and Black, T. G. (2010). Life outside the 50-minute hour: The personal lives of counsellors. *Canadian Journal of Counselling and Psychotherapy*, 44, 421–437. https://cjc-rcc.ucalgary.ca/article/view/59243

Kernberg, O. F. (1975). *Borderline Conditions and Pathological Narcissism.* New York: Jason Aronson.

Kinet, M. (2023). *The Spirit of the Drive in Neuropsychoanalysis.* London/New York: Routledge.

Kinet, M. (2024). *Psychoanalytic Principles in Psychiatric Practice. A Remedy by Truth.* London/New York: Routledge.

Klasen, J., Nolte, T., Möller, H., and Taubner, S. (2019). Aversive Kindheitserfahrungen, Bindungsrepräsentationen und Mentalisierungsfähigkeit von Psychotherapeuten in Ausbildung. *Zeitschrift für Psychosomatische Medizin und Psychotherapie*, 65 (4). doi:10.13109/zptm.2019.65.4.353

Klein, M. (1935). A contribution to the psychogenesis of manic-depressive states. *Love, Guilt and Reparation and Other Works 1921–1945* (pp. 262–289). London: Hogarth, 1975.

Klein, M. (1946). Notes on some schizoid mechanisms. *Envy and Gratitude and Other Works 1946–1963* (pp. 1–24). London: Hogarth, 1975.

Klein, M. (1957). Envy and gratitude. *Envy and gratitude and other works 1946–1963* (pp. 176–235). London: Virago, 1988.

Lacan, J. (1957–1958/). *Le Séminaire, Livre V: Les formations de l'inconscient* (J.-A. Miller, ed.). Paris: Seuil, 1998.

Lacan, J. (1959–1960). *The Seminar of Jacques Lacan, Book VII: The Ethics of Psychoanalysis, 1959–1960* (D. Porter, trans.). New York: Norton, 1992.

Lacan, J. (1962–1963). *Le Séminaire, Livre X: L'angoisse* (J.-A. Miller, ed.). Paris: Seuil, 2004.

Laverdière, O., Kealy, D., Ogrodniczuk, J. S., Chamberland, S., and Descôteaux, J. (2019). Psychotherapists' professional quality of life. *Traumatology*, 25, 208–215.

Lemma, A. (2015). *Introduction to the Practice of Psychoanalytic Psychotherapy.* New York: Wiley.

Levy, K. N., Meehan, K. B., Kelly, K. M., Reynoso, J. S., Weber, M., Clarkin, J. F., and Kernberg, O. F. (2006). Change in attachment patterns and reflective function in a randomized control trial of transference-focused psychotherapy for borderline personality disorder. *Journal of Consulting and Clinical Psychology*, 74 (6), 1027–1040.

Lingiardi, V., and McWilliams, N. (2018). Introduction to the special issue on the Psychodynamic Diagnostic Manual, (PDM-2): The PDM: Yesterday, today, tomorrow. *Psychoanalytic Psychology*, 35 (3), 289. doi:10.1037/pap0000188

Luborsky, L., Crits-Christoph, P., McLellan, A. T., Woody, G., Piper, W., Liberman, B., Imber, S., and Pilkonis, P. (1986). Do therapists vary much in their success? Findings from four outcome studies. *American Journal of Orthopsychiatry*, 56 (4), 501–512.

Malach-Pines, A., and Yafe-Yenai, O. (1999). Unconscious influences on a choice of career: implications for organizational consultation. *Journal of Health and Human Services Administration*, 21 (4), 502–511.

Maroda, K. J. (2022). *The Analyst's Vulnerability: Impact on Theory and Practice.* London/New York: Routledge.

Masiran, N. A., Ibrahim, N., Nik Jaafar, N. R., and Siau, C. S. (2023). The positive and negative aspects of parentification: An integrated review. *Frontiers in Psychology*, 14, 1159739. doi:10.1016/j.childyouth.2022.106709

Masson, J. M. (ed. and trans.). (1985). *The Complete Letters of Sigmund Freud to Wilhelm Fliess, 1887–1904*. Cambridge, MA: Harvard University Press.

McWilliams, N. (2004). *Psychoanalytic Psychotherapy: A Practitioner's Guide.* New York: Guilford.

Miller, A. (1979). *The Drama of the Gifted Child: The Search for the True Self* (3rd edn). New York: Basic Books, 2008.

Mintz, D. L. (2015). Teaching the prescriber's role: The psychology of psychopharmacology. *Academic Psychiatry*, 29 (2), 187–194. doi:10.1176/appi.ap.29.2.187

Murphy, R. A., and Halgin, R. P. (1995). Influences on the career choice of psychotherapists. *Professional Psychology: Research and Practice*, 26, 422–425.

Norcross, J. C., and Farber, B. A. (2005). Choosing psychotherapy as a career: Beyond 'I want to help people.' *Journal of Clinical Psychology*, 61 (8), 939–943. doi:10.1002/jclp.20175

Norcross, J. C., and VandenBos, G. R. (2018). *Leaving it at the Office: A Guide to Psychotherapist Self-Care.* New York: Guilford.

Orlinsky, D. E., and Rønnestad, M. H. (2005). *How Psychotherapists Develop: A Study of Therapeutic Work and Professional Growth.* Washington, DC: American Psychological Association.

Panksepp, J. (1998). *Affective Neuroscience: The Foundations of Human and Animal Emotions.* Oxford: Oxford University Press.

Phillips, A. (1993). *On Kissing, Tickling, and Being Bored: Psychoanalytic Essays on the Unexamined Life.* Cambridge, MA: Harvard University Press.

Phillips, A. (2007). *Winnicott.* London: Penguin Books.

Råbu, M., Moltu, C., Binder, P. E., and McLeod, J. (2016). How does practicing psychotherapy affect the personal life of the therapist? A qualitative inquiry of senior therapists' experiences. *Psychotherapy Research*, 26 (6), 737–749. doi:10.1080/10503307.2015.1065354

Rek, I., Ehrenthal, J. C., Strauss, B. M., Schauenburg, H., Nikendei, C. and Dinger, U. (2018). Attachment styles and interpersonal motives of psychotherapy trainees. *Psychotherapy*, 55 (3), 209–215.

Smith, P. L., and Moss, S. B. (2009). Psychologist impairment: What is it, how can it be prevented, and what can be done to address it? *Clinical Psychology: Science and Practice*, 16, 1–15. https://psycnet.apa.org/doi/10.1111/j.1468-2850.2009.01137.x

Solms, M. (2021). *The Hidden Spring: A Journey to the Source of Consciousness*. New York: Norton.

Staal, C. (2024). De psychotherapeut als wounded healer. *De Psycholoog*. April, pp. 11–18. https://www.tijdschriftdepsycholoog.nl/wetenschap/de-psychotherapeut-als-wounded-healer/

Steele, M., Kaniuk, J., Hodges, J, Asquith, K., Hillmann, and Steele, H. (2008). Measuring mentalization across contexts. In E. Jurist, A. Slade, and S. Bergner (eds), *Mind to Mind: Infant Research, Neuroscience and Psychoanalysis* (pp. 115–139). New York: Other Press.

Sussman, M. B. (1992). *A Curious Calling. Unconscious Motivations for Practising Psychotherapy*. Northvale, NJ; London: Jason Aronson.

Van Gael, M. (1998). Als de chirurg in eigen vingers snijdt. Over de grenzen van de draagkracht van de psychotherapeut. *Tijdschrift voor Psychotherapie*, 24, 28–35.

Van Gael, M. (2000). Is de therapeut 'vrij van herinnering en verlangen?' *Tijdschrift Klinische Psychologie*, 30 (1), 4–12.

Van Gael, M. (2020). Als de chirurg in eigen vingers snijdt – anno 2020. *Tijdschrift voor Psychotherapie*, 46 (3), 151–164.

West, M. L., and Keller, A. E. (1991). Parentification of the child: A case study of Bowlby's compulsive care-giving attachment pattern. *American Journal of Psychotherapy*, 45 (3), 425–431.

Winer, J. (1994). The parentified therapist. *Contemporary Psychoanalysis*, 30 (2), 297–314.

Winnicott, D. W. (1958). The capacity to be alone. *International Journal of Psycho-Analysis*, 39, 416–420.

Winnicott, D. W. (1960). The theory of the parent-infant relationship. *International Journal of Psycho-Analysis*, 41, 585–595.

Winnicott, D. W. (1965). *The Maturational Processes and the Facilitating Environment: Studies in the Theory of Emotional Development*. London: Hogarth.

Winnicott, D. W. (1971). *Playing and Reality*. London: Tavistock.

Wrzesniewski, A., McCauley, C., Rozin, P., and Schwartz, B. (1997). Jobs, careers, and callings: People's relations to their work. *Journal of Research in Personality*, 31(1), 21–33.

Zerubavel, N., and Wright, M. O. (2012). The dilemma of the wounded healer. *Psychotherapy*, 49 (4), 482–491.

Žižek, S. (1992). *Enjoy Your Symptom! Jacques Lacan in Hollywood and Out*. London/New York: Routledge.

Chapter 12

Intermezzo V

The Parentified Psychotherapist

In this intermezzo, I sketch three portraits in which parentification figures in the psychotherapeutic vocation.

Margot is in her forties, lives with John, is the mother of a son and a daughter, and works as a psychologist in a group GP practice. She comes for consultation because her colleague is travelling around the States for a few months. She was dreading it because she couldn't imagine coping without him. She felt very abandoned and only now realises how emotionally dependent she has become on him. When she thinks about it, she realises that this happens quite often. 'Unconsciously, I make myself dependent. I seek protection from a father figure. Maybe I missed that in the past.' She promptly adds: 'But that says nothing about my relationship with my husband!'

The first conversation is often like an opera overture. Many later themes and motifs are announced. Both the patient and the therapist only realise the full significance of the words spoken at that time after a while. She immediately makes it clear that she is not seeking an extramarital relationship. She senses that it is about past hurts. She has missed a lot and kept quiet about much of it. She describes her parents as hardworking, understanding, and gentle. But they never saw what she was carrying with her and what weighed on the family. Margot first talks about a court case that dragged on for many years. Her parents suffered greatly from it, and she could see that they were giving up. Margot wanted to spare them her 'shit.' She put herself last. She made her plan mentally. Practically and logistically, her parents were there, but they didn't notice anything unusual about Margot. Her mother now feels terrible that she knew nothing, but she can't blame her. 'I always kept everything to myself!' Then there is the older sister, Katie, who did not exactly welcome Margot. She was jealous of her presence. Her parents never noticed anything, even though Katie humiliated her on a daily basis. Katie hit her, locked her up, threatened her with a knife and was also physically abusive at times. Her sister had a big mouth and attracted a lot of care and attention. Margot herself never did anything wrong and lovingly cared for her younger

DOI: 10.4324/9781003645726-12

brother. 'I was very well-behaved.' As a child, she dreamed of having an older brother who could protect her.

John is slightly older and is a foreman at his workplace. It took him a long time to want to get married, but they have now been married for over ten years. Margot says they have a good relationship, but her husband does not want to have psychological conversations: 'I am not your patient!' He is rather quiet and closed off and retreats to the garden shed every day, where he has been smoking cannabis for years. He comes from a difficult home situation. His parents are divorced, his brother took his own life, and he felt rejected and abandoned. 'He's a bottler; misery has kept us together! John realises what I mean to him!'

She goes on to say that during her teenage years, she fell asleep crying almost every night. She felt alone and abandoned. Those feelings still surface often, 'even though everything is fine now.' She describes her father as a hard-working, sensitive man who owned a horticultural business. He was always terrorised and pushed around by her mother. Margot's mother always remained strong and courageous. She had to keep things running and was constantly busy. Following an industrial accident with multiple victims, her father was held legally responsible. After a gruelling legal battle, he was ultimately ordered to pay very high damages, which nearly bankrupted them. Margot knew everything, but was not allowed to talk to anyone about it. 'I wanted to be a solicitor at first!' Her father also talked about suicide when he was alone with Margot. He was planning to hang himself. Margot was always the one who listened. She listened to her mother, too. While her sister was very present and loud, Margot preferred to stay in the background. Regarding further information on her development, she was very popular in nursery school. She was anxious, though. 'I didn't dare do a somersault,' she tells me. In primary school, she was always top of the class. She was bullied by other pupils because of this. In secondary school, she hardly had to study and still achieved excellent results, while Katy had to work very hard to get through her technical education. Margot kept a low profile among her peers. She had very pale skin and was laughed at for it. She was sad because she wanted to do right by everyone. She remembers well a strict piano teacher who constantly criticised her and also tapped her fingers hard. She literally developed balance problems, causing her to fall several times. After two years of commuting, she moved into student accommodation during her psychology studies. She felt very lonely and socially inept. For years, she was in love with a friend's older brother. She cherished his concern and care. In recent years, she has been seeing a psychotherapist infrequently, but she feels she has been cheating. 'I just sold her some psychobabble.'

Margot came for weekly face-to-face psychotherapy sessions for two years. I got to know her as an extremely caring and responsible, as well as very compassionate, psychologist who was always ready to take on difficult therapeutic tasks. She often let herself be taken advantage of by people who acted like nurses and had difficulty setting boundaries for her 24/7 caregiving nature. Her relationship with her partner came under particular scrutiny. In the transference, John was more like the distressed father who lacked sufficient resilience and leaned on her. He had been medically unfit for work for a long time (reportedly due to burnout) and she feared that sooner or later he would cause a traffic accident under the influence, with all the legal/financial consequences that would entail. Eventually, she got him to see a psychotherapist, with whom he has now built up a relationship and from whom he is apparently beginning to learn to talk. Occasionally, he now opens his mouth instead of retreating to his garden shed to let off steam. This allows her to relinquish her psychological role (at least within the relationship) and stand up more for her own interests as a woman and as a mother.

During his first analysis, Sebastian lay on the couch three times a week for five years. The reason for this was that, after completing his training as a specialist in psychiatry, a nun who was the director of his training centre had promised him a good job as a manager in a psychiatric hospital. He had even moved to another region for this, but in extremis, a candidate with familial ties was chosen instead in an act of nepotism. This left him feeling lost, while his wife was getting off to a flying start in the same sector.

Sebastian is an only child. As the eldest of seven, his father had really wanted a large family, but this proved unfeasible for his mother for medical reasons. Although they did their best, both pedagogically and materially, to avoid all the dangers of the cliché of a spoiled only child, Sebastian felt emotionally caught between two magnifying glasses. Against his will (and that of his parents), he was a walking hot spot. His mother stayed at home to look after her 'darling' until he started nursery school. At that time, his father was often away for long periods of time due to professional assignments abroad. However, when he was at home, he was also completely crazy about his son. At first glance, the nursery school period went smoothly. However, after the first term of the first year of primary school, Sebastian suddenly found himself at the bottom of the class. He went from hero to zero, as it were. He was terribly panicked and lay awake at night worrying about it. The result: for the rest of that school year and the following ones, he was *primus perpetuus*—or, in other words, *nulli secundus*, second to none. In the sixth year, he was even first in all subjects/in all areas. This top-student pattern only ended around the age of sixteen. Puberty and adolescence simply establish a different pecking order than school grades do. The latter are not very sexy. He tried, with limited success, to become a lady-killer and mainly fell in love platonically or set his sights on slightly older girls. At home, meanwhile, he had always been exemplary and well-behaved, making the beds, vacuuming, setting the table and, by the time his parents came home from work, placing their slippers at the top of the stairs so that they only had to slip their feet into them. His mother was often overworked and stressed, so he didn't want to be a burden to her. She complained a lot about the tyranny of her bosses, Mr. D. and Mr. V.

During his father's absences, Sebastian behaved like an obedient conversation partner. He described his mother as a very emotional, if not theatrical, figure; he felt he was the apple of her eye but also her confidant. Father was much more reserved: a man of few words. They often went out together for all kinds of sporting activities and adventures. Father was noticeably struggling with ulcerative colitis (in the form of pain and frequent urgent visits to the toilet) and was undergoing homoeopathic treatment for this. He would have liked to have become a general practitioner himself and was (partly for this reason) an ardent fan of Anton Chekhov and W. Somerset Maugham. Sebastian was also very upset that his father had to go to therapy. His mother told him that his father cried loudly at a kind of primal scream therapist about his mother, who had died in her last cot. Sebastian was sad and angry because of what he saw as a particularly humiliating approach.

During that phase of his life, he had a recurring dream. In it, he had to walk for miles along a high, narrow wall. He felt that the well-being and survival of the two peoples living on either side depended on his maintaining his balance. Naturally, this dream was discussed at length in his therapy. First of all, Sebastian was not only a golden boy, but he also had a double Oedipus complex. In the early days, he felt like the man of the house. In nursery school, he had to be repeatedly reprimanded for making excessive demands on what was going on under his classmates' skirts. In a second phase, he adored his father and hated his mother to the point of murder. At night, for example, he would lie awake, furious at her hissing 's' as she talked to his father in the adjoining bedroom. He associated this with the s of serpent and talked about his mother's Es (Freud's German for the Id). During puberty, he suffered two boxing fractures (metacarpal V) by punching a wall with his fist. The first time was because he was being harassed by a friend who repeatedly disrupted his time with a girlfriend at the time, and the second time was during one of the many heated conflicts with his father during his final years of high school. The dream of the 'Chinese' wall turned out (as is often the case with recurring dreams) to be the story of his life. Throughout his career, integration between very diverse visions or perspectives seemed to be a matter of life and death, as it were. It involved a sustained balancing act that was apparently vital to him for a smooth course and a good outcome. He maintained a high level of integration, but this resulted in a rather isolated position. For example, he published too literary for academics and too academic for literary figures; his therapeutic approach was too psychiatric for psychoanalysts and too psychoanalytical for psychiatrists; and his theoretical inspiration was too Lacanian for non-Lacanians and not Lacanian enough for Lacanians. The rescue fantasy that emerges from the dream was rooted, on the one hand, in feelings of guilt about both matricidal and patricidal impulses. If you want to be *numero uno*, all competition must be beaten or defeated. In addition to his tendency towards *Wiedergutmachung* or reparation, he had read between the lines about his parents' difficulties and felt called upon to alleviate their divergent needs/desires. A commonly used abbreviation for psychoanalysis is, incidentally, PA. For Sebastian, it was not only a calling but also a symptom and a passion. In his biography of Freud, Peter Gay refers to psychoanalysis more specifically as a *tender passion*. Sebastian also takes a stand against the denial or disregard of psychological suffering in society. Some, therefore, regard psychoanalysis as the political party for psychiatric patients. Sebastian often let slip the remark: 'If I were Minister of Health…!'

Sylvia is a psychologist and initially came to me for her training therapy. She has worked in various psychiatric hospitals and is in an LAT relationship with Maxwell, a general practitioner of her age. She is the eldest of three and has two younger brothers. Her father is a highly educated executive in the IT sector. He was recently diagnosed with ASD. Her mother was recently undergoing psychiatric treatment. Sylvia initially referred to her as a borderline patient, although she now wonders whether ASD may also be a factor in her case. Both of her younger brothers are single. They live together in her parents' flat and, according to her, are not coping very well. The eldest is a paramedic and the youngest is a logistics employee in a hospital. Sylvia always appears cheerful and smiling, but behind this façade lie depression and a great deal of abandonment anxiety. This time, I will limit myself to an anthology of a few verbatim quotes from her weekly psychotherapy sessions.

> Our home wasn't decorated. It was all empty space. There were no photos of family members or of us. As a child, I found that sad. My friends had photos like that. They were proud to show them off. At our house, everything was sterile. We also had to wash our hands constantly. There were all kinds of strange rules. For example, we had to sort our rubbish very strictly. My father's autism made him very meticulous. How we had to wash saucers. How we had to stack them in the cupboard. My housemate can also get very angry if I put something in the wrong place. Such comments have the same impact as before.
>
> I had to be very kind to my brothers. I did that too. I took care of them. I protected them. If their swimming trunks were pulled off in the swimming pool, I was the tough one who fought for them. My parents didn't do any of that for me. My parents never played with us. My mother always made me play with my brothers. As the first grandchild, I was my grandfather's favourite. My mother couldn't stand that. She had been neglected in comparison to her sister. That aunt likes to read books. She is exuberant, sweet and sociable. She is also coquettish and feminine. She wears low-cut dresses. I like that, but my mother always reacts curtly and jealously.
>
> My mother is always reproachful. She also constantly wants recognition. That irritates me. She's like a whining adult woman. She wants to cook at every family gathering. She ruins everything with her strange, alternative creations. We all eat reluctantly, and meanwhile, she nags:

'You don't want my food.' And then I supposedly had eating problems as a child! I just didn't like her cooking. I wasn't allowed to season my food. She saw this as an insult. The food was always bland and tasteless. Sometimes it made me gag, but it was just like thickened water. Not pleasant. She focused mainly on healthy eating. She constantly commented that I was too thin, but she made things I didn't like. She forced me to eat spoonfuls of margarine. What mother does that? She might as well have given me a feeding tube, I think now. When we went to play with other children, we were allowed to eat pancakes with our hands. At home, that was not allowed. Always those table manners. I often dream of a pale ghost or a frightened kitten scratching, and on the other side of a cute little blond boy. By now, I am sure that they refer to my mother and father, respectively.

My father-in-law is seriously ill. Still, he wants to help us move, but my mother has to go to some woolly workshop again. I would like to be vicious, but that's pointless. It takes effort to swallow my annoyance. I limit contact with my mother. I talk about trivial matters. I had nightmares for a long time after a family party. Now I mainly feel a sense of loss. I have no parental bond whatsoever. It's completely the opposite.

Every time I change jobs, I find it very difficult to let go. I put a lot of effort into calming the team (of a unit for personality disorders). There was a lot of aggressive behaviour from both patients and the team. The psychiatrist, Dr V, was often absent. She sees me as her extension. She barely takes me into account. I don't think she's ever been in therapy herself. She has narcissistic tendencies, takes everything personally, is easily offended and rather dominant. It seems I always have to have it at least as hard as she does. She thinks it's obvious that I should spend all my energy filling her shoes. She's just like one of those Knokke dolls: dressed up and Botoxed. She doesn't see it in herself, but she's cynical and rigid. I wouldn't want to be like that. It's the same with Mum, of course. She doesn't go to therapy either. I want to set my priorities differently. I want to live my own life more; my motherhood and my own children definitely take precedence. My mother, Dr V… how much effort do I have to put into pleasing her? Afterwards, I think: fuck you! Dr V is a real shrew.

Maxwell and I want to buy a house together. Right now, I share an apartment with my brothers. They don't take good care of themselves or the apartment. Do I have to be the protective older sister again? Rubbish is piling up in their room. I also have a lot of paperwork at the solicitors. It's a huge pile of abstract documents and certificates. My brothers are supposed to email things, but they just don't. They say they don't have time. Meanwhile, our parents aren't helping at all. I try to stick to my role as big sister. It bothers me that they don't take responsibility. Of course, we had a different upbringing. I always took care of things, and they ran away from difficult situations. I feel pity and annoyance. I don't want to be responsible for anyone in my family anymore! It irritates me enormously that they are all dysfunctional. At first, I didn't notice it with my brothers, but neither of them finished their studies. I used to think they were emotionally mature, but now they are stuck. We used to have an alliance: pulling together against our difficult parents. I also used to look up to a friend, but she has now developed anorexia and borderline personality disorder. I used to think people had personality, but not anymore. For a long time, I also thought my mother was normal. I didn't find her warm, though. As a child, there was a lot of sadness. For example, Mummy never took me anywhere. Not to the playground, not to the zoo, not to an amusement park. She spent a lot of time in bed. I didn't like that. I think I only realised that something was seriously wrong with her during my internships. I have always been ashamed of my parents. Now I look at them as if they were puppets. I don't like it, but I no longer feel compelled to constantly clean up their mess.

Chapter 13

The Psychodynamics and Psychogenesis of Parentification

Introduction

In describing parentification, we began with family therapists. They work with children who are still growing up and obviously need to involve the child's environment in the treatment. Through projective identification, a bridge was built to the inner world of the parent and how they can keep the child under their spell. Now we will focus more on what is going on in the child's mind. However, we will mainly draw on our psychotherapeutic work with *adults*. As described elsewhere, we systematically seek to integrate psychiatry and psychoanalysis.[1] Patterns of parentification have been imprinted in adults' implicit or procedural memory. Patients cannot remember them, but they are expressed in repetition and in (inter)action. They are decisive for how they relate to their environment and for how they appear live on stage, both outside and within the total transference situation of the treatment relationship or environment. In this way, they can be (re)constructively and psychotherapeutically processed.

Despite its clinical relevance, parentification is somewhat neglected in psychoanalytic theory. It is sometimes mentioned in passing in connection with rescuer fantasies, narcissistic pathology, or False Self problems, which usually conceal unintegrated and unmentalised content relating to abandonment, anger, and depression. Parentification can be the result of (psycho)pathology in the parent(s). It can go hand in hand with (and is in itself a form of) trauma. Certain major life events (death, illness, divorce) can cause developmental interference, which may be accompanied by a factor of parentification. Finally, it can be a pathogenetic element in neurotic, narcissistic, and borderline problems in the patient.

We will first briefly formulate a few basic principles concerning the so-called neoteny, or neurophysiological and other immaturities, that are so characteristic of human children. After all, it results in a whole period of absolute dependence on the Big Other. We simply need sufficient nourishment and upbringing in order to develop optimally.[2] Problems during this period can lead to the development of a False Self. This is the deeper ground in

DOI: 10.4324/9781003645726-13

which parentification can already take root. The individuation-separation phase is also an important milestone. Can/may the child go its own way at all? What inevitable tensions result from the Lacanian mirror stage and the register of the imaginary that is based on it? We will then examine the (also early) Oedipus complex and zoom in on castration and the phallus in particular. First, we will outline a constellation in which parentification can play a role.

Dependency

Due to our physiological immaturity, we are absolutely dependent on the Big Other from birth. This first Big Other is usually the mother: Big (M)Other. She must respond to our distress ('*Schmerz*') through what Freud calls a 'specific action.'[3] This involves countless micro-moments in which the mother (imaginatively) mirrors and (symbolically) marks. If she provides this care adequately, a kind of atmosphere forms around the newborn child. Freud and Bion call this a stimulus shield, while Didier Anzieu speaks of a skin-ego or '*moi-peau*.'[4] The mother continuously weaves this protective blanket for her child.[5] If the small child is deprived of such mentalising responsiveness, this can have catastrophic consequences on a psychological level: unspeakable shivers, threats of destruction, or unthinkable fear can occur and leave deep craters in the psyche.[6]

Various vital abilities develop with sufficient encouragement during early childhood. It is necessary for the establishment of secure attachment, for the development of mentalising ability and reflective functioning.[7] These are, in fact, the most important protective factors for later (psycho)pathology. These fundamental processes between the young child and the mother (environment) are also decisive for drive and affect regulation. They contribute to self- and object constancy. They are essential for the establishment of a narcissistic balance and for the development of a True and cohesive Self, and they play a major role in the acquisition of (gender) identity and sexual orientation.

Parentification can already result from problems at this basic level. The Big Other (e.g., due to personality, condition, or situation) is overly preoccupied with their own needs, wants, and dependence. This results in reduced sensitivity, emotional availability, attunement, or mirroring.[8] The mother does not respond to the child's needs; rather, it is the child who tries to respond to the mother's needs. This creates a double problem for the child: lack and excess. Excess because the child has to bear the burden of the Other (it tries, as it were, to be a protective blanket for the mother) and lack because the child is not sufficiently nourished with vital illusions such as safety and security. The play space is also insufficiently open. The presence and absence of the mother are not symbolically mediated. Normally, the child develops, so to speak, an endoskeleton. This provides inner consistency. However, when security is lacking, an exoskeleton develops instead. The child is protected (like an insect) against extreme harmful stimuli. However, inside or behind this shield, it remains soft and underdeveloped. All this corresponds, of course, to some of Winnicott's descriptions.[9] According to him, the True Self forms the core of the person. It develops thanks to a (maternal) environment that allows itself to be found and discovered by responding spontaneously to the child. In the absence of this, the environment is not safe but threatening. The child develops a False Self as a defence. This Self can also be a narcissistic or grandiose bastion, as in Otto Kernberg's theory.[10]

We can compare it to imaginary defence mechanisms that we share with animals that defend themselves against their predators. When fight or flight are not possible, only freezing and defeat remain. Behind this 'mask' or armour, a True Self remains, but it is impoverished. The 'capacity to be alone' (where one is forgotten 'in the presence of the mother') has not been able to develop sufficiently.[11] This capacity involves a trusting surrender to the mother and a state of non-integration, in which the child can be both 'naked' and 'at ease.' Instead, it is vigilant. In contemporary terms, it may develop an avoidant or preoccupied attachment style, for example.[12] In the first case, it is quiet, easily exemplary and causes the Other neither trouble nor inconvenience. In the second case, it tries not only to spare the Other but also to appease them. The child is hypersensitive to the Other's needs and other sources of discomfort, which it tries to alleviate as much as possible to create a safe mother environment for itself.

When the child enters the individuation-separation phase[13] and literally and figuratively leaves the mother, it constantly looks back. It fears not only that maternal support will disappear, but also—and above all—that the mother will not accept its departure. The child asks itself the following question, so to speak: is it right for me to show that my mother is not indispensable? After all, the child believes it must satisfy its mother's narcissistic or oral needs in order to retain or win her love. Conversely, it is threatened with abandonment or destruction if it does not desire to satisfy its mother's wishes. This can be recognised, for example, in patients who behave more like a mirror and an echo than a real conversation partner. This creates a claustrophobic anxiety that causes fear, but also triggers feelings of anger and hatred that must be suppressed. After all, the child must above all make the Other feel good. Such an Other is both dominant and overwhelming as well as weak and vulnerable. A thick cloak of love and care is needed to suppress repressed feelings of anger and hatred (even murderous tendencies) and to remove them from view and consciousness.

Dependence, on the other hand, is a narcissistic injury. It sometimes makes us 'hate to love.' The Other embodies the Ideal Self, seems whole and self-satisfied, without lack. The contrast with the child's helplessness or fragmentation is great. For Lacan, the mirror stage therefore contains an inseparable aggressive component that (as we shall see) is missing in attachment theory.[14] The child wants to be this all-good and all-powerful object. That is why it is also hated and must be destroyed. For the Kleinians, this aggressive component takes on mythical proportions and is considered constitutionally determined envy.[15] When the child reaches the depressive position or 'the stage of concern,' it wants to make amends for the damage it has caused and repair it.[16] From a Kleinian perspective, this repair forms the core of both love and creativity.[17] This is how parentification can initially represent a reparative compromise solution to conflicts surrounding aggressive impulses for the child.

Oedipus Complex

But the child is not only absolutely dependent on the mother for its survival. It is also dependent on the mother's *love*. This mother appears and disappears according to a rationale that is obscure and enigmatic to the child.[18] For the child, it is her will and whim that is law, and the child feels totally and fatally at the mercy of this '*loi de caprice*.'[19] As in '*Les yeux de ma mère*,' the famous chanson by Arno: '*Ma mère, elle a quelque chose. Quelque chose dangereuse. Quelque chose d'une allumeuse. Quelque chose d'une emmerdeuse*.'[20] Moreover, the child feels all too keenly that the mother seems to desire something or someone other than constantly satisfying the child. The child tries to identify with the imaginary object of her desire. It tries to be everything to her or (as it is called) her phallus. This phallus should not be confused with the fickle body part that half of humanity possesses. On the one hand, it is imaginary: the hypothetical (because non-existent) don't know *what*/'*je ne sais quoi*' that could completely satisfy the mother. On the other hand, it is symbolic: a signifier given by the father. In Paul Verhaeghe's famous formulation, it is that which we can never have or be enough of to satisfy desire or fill the void of the Other.[21] From a cultural perspective, in Lacanian thought, the phallus is the privileged signifier around which differences and values are organised. As such, it represents power and authority within the symbolic order.

Lacan distinguishes between three logical (rather than chronological) stages of the Oedipus complex. For him, the mother-child relationship is never a dual relationship, even though it does lead to a duel. Who has the power? Who rules the roost? Who owns the phallus? From the outset, Lacan sees the mother-child relationship as triangular. This concerns the early Oedipus with mother and child, and, as a third term, the phallus.[22] The child experiences successive frustrations because of a mother who desires *elsewhere*/'*qui* désire ailleurs.' It wants to be everything its mother desires. The (imaginary) father then castrates ('privation') the mother first, denying her *jouissance* (which in a legal context literally means usufruct) of the child. Finally, the (real) father will castrate the child, so that it can no longer be everything/the phallus of the mother. This 'last' period is castration in the narrower sense. It protects the child from the desire of the devouring, omnipotent mother to whom it would otherwise be defencelessly surrendered.[23] We recognise in this the rotten calling in which we lose ourselves and to which we would succumb. It is absolutely necessary that the paternal function puts a stop to this (the phallus).

This is implicit in a well-known statement by Françoise Dolto: that, for the child's development, the parents' love for each other is more important than the parents' love for the child.[24] If the parents have an unsatisfactory relationship, a skewed triangle can arise, in which one or both parents seek satisfaction from the child. The child is thus not sufficiently exposed to loving parents in a sexual couple. They seem to be more attached to their mother and/or father than to their partner and think they can or must satisfy their desires. The boundaries between the sexes, between the generations and those relating to the prohibition of incest become unclear. The child who is thus parentified by the parent(s) is also increasingly abandoned by the other parent. What is lacking is the paternal function, which, as a third term, must both prohibit and protect. Normally, it curbs the boundless love in which parent and child merge in a sick or deadly way in that mixture of pain and pleasure that Lacan calls *jouissance*.

But let me first discuss the panoply of psychoanalytic perspectives one by one. We will start chronologically with Freud and logically end with Lacan. After all, many pre-Oedipal components that are decisive for parentification play out within their respective frameworks.

Sigmund Freud: Some Relevant Concepts

Although Freud himself never used the term parentification, a number of his metapsychological insights into narcissism, object choice, the Oedipus complex, identification, and trauma already provide a fruitful framework for understanding these psychodynamics. Indeed, his work repeatedly lays the foundation for later psychoanalytic approaches to reversed care relationships and their consequences. In an earlier book, I therefore referred to Freud as the fountainhead.[25]

In his introduction to narcissism, Freud distinguishes between two fundamental forms of object choice: the anaclitic (supportive) and the narcissistic.[26] In reality, it is always a certain combination of both. In the first, love objects are chosen modelled on the first caregivers, while in the second, the object is chosen in one's own image and likeness (as we see ourselves: now, in the past, or ideally). In the first case, the parents' early childhood/oral needs are central. This is when a parent uses a child primarily as a mirror, as a source of confirmation, or to support a fragile sense of self (worth), based on narcissistic wounds. In both cases, the child is not loved for who they are, but for how they make the parent feel (about themselves). In this dynamic, the child is used to regulate the parent's own (narcissistic or otherwise) balance. The price is high: the child's own needs are suppressed, and the development of an autonomous self is hindered by the parent's need for appreciation.

Freud's Oedipus complex is often understood too narrowly as purely sexual, whereas it is mainly about triangulation and how the child navigates between roles and boundaries.[27] In its typical form, the child desires exclusive love from one parent and (therefore) rivals the other parent. This results in identification with one or the other parent and the letting go of incestuous desires. This logic is disrupted or reversed in parentification. A parent may unconsciously seduce the child into a partner-like relationship, thus creating a skewed rather than a straight triangle. This results in a Pyrrhic victory for the child, as the triumph leads to guilt and punishment, including lifelong loyalty to the rival parent figure. Emotional incest violates not so much the sexual taboo as the generational distinction between parent and child. The parent uses the child as an emotional partner, and the child confuses love with care and responsibility.

In his text on the ego and mass psychology, Freud described identification as the first form of emotional bond.[28] The child unconsciously identifies with certain characteristics of the object rather than entering into a relationship with it. This identification forms the core of the ego and later of the superego. However, when a child grows up in a context of parentification, it does not identify with the parent as a role model, but with the parent's ego ideal. The child thus strongly internalises the parent's desire to be a saviour or morally superior, and develops a False Self that is focused on pleasing and repairing. The child's ego organises itself around serving, pleasing, or rescuing the parent at the expense of its own spontaneity, assertiveness or pleasure. The resulting distortion of the superego leads to chronic feelings of guilt and an excessive sense of responsibility. The child's own needs evoke anxiety, and there is an inability to legitimise them for itself. It is a precursor to Winnicott's False Self: the identification with an ideal that overshadows one's own spontaneity.[29] The natural desires of the child (dependence, play, neediness) are therefore often experienced as weakness or a burden in parentification.

Around the same time, Freud came to understand trauma as an excess of excitement that overwhelms the ability to bond with symbolic-imaginary representations.[30] From this perspective, emotional parentification can also be understood as the child 'binding' the parental chaos, serving as a stimulus shield. In that case, all negative feelings are covered by the proverbial cloak of love.

Freud himself described another intriguing variant of parentification in adult love: the man who is repeatedly attracted to prostitutes or women with a bad sexual reputation out of a desire to save them.[31] Freud interprets this saviour fantasy as a repetition of an Oedipal dynamic. At first, the boy sees his mother as a saint and cannot accept what she does with his father in the bedroom. He becomes jealous and resents his mother for betraying him. The result: the desire arises to save the mother and thus win her back, or to transform the 'whore-like' mother back into the idyllic Madonna.[32] For Freud, these saviour fantasies are a detour to repeat forbidden desires without acknowledging them. They are narcissistically coloured because the saviour seeks to repair his own brokenness in the other person.

All these psychodynamics can recur in what contemporary authors call the *Florence Nightingale syndrome.*[33] People with this tendency define themselves through caring for others. Paula Lampe refers to this as *the Mother Teresa syndrome*: they collect wretches like stamps. In *the White Knight syndrome*, American psychologists Lamia and Krieger describe how such rescuers often fall in love with vulnerable partners in order to feel valuable through them. Slaying other people's dragons is their *raison d'être.* As soon as the partner is cured or becomes independent, the tension disappears, and they look for a new person in need to rescue.[34] The need to help has, as it were, become an addiction. It provides narcissistic satisfaction, but masks a lack of self-esteem. The rescuer projects his need for affirmation onto the other person and denies his dependence. The therapist thus becomes a victim of his own urge to help. Further on, the phenomenon of *compulsive caregiving* is discussed as a defensive strategy described by John Bowlby that arises in childhood: the child learns that love and appreciation can only be obtained by caring for others.[35] This caregiving function is internalised as a survival mechanism, a form of conditional self-esteem. This dynamic can be particularly prevalent in the helping professions. Freud already warned against the '*furor sanandi*,' the healing instinct that can blind the analyst to the patient's autonomy.[36] In this context, Manfred Kets de Vries refers to the *rescuer syndrome*, which is often ridiculed in romantic relationships (even by 'laypeople').[37] Although seemingly driven to comfort the unhappy woman, the lover is out to exploit her vulnerability. The greater her grief, the more powerful/potent he feels himself to be. The prince on the white horse (or nowadays: in the white convertible) is essentially a sinister hero. When such rescuers base their identity too strongly on helping, they lose their boundaries. The danger is a collusion in which the therapist takes on the role of parent and the patient that of dependent child, resulting in repetition rather than interpretation.

Sándor Ferenczi: From Trauma to Technique

Freud himself paid relatively little attention to the pre-Oedipal mother-child relationship. With his *retour à Freud*,[38] Lacan in particular would remain 'faithful' to Freud's Oedipal logic, in which certain issues such as castration, the paternal function, and the Name/No of the Father remain at the zenith.[39] However, the first generation of psychoanalysts, such as Karl Abraham, Otto Rank, and, above all, Sándor Ferenczi, resolutely placed the (early) mother-child relationship at the forefront. In an earlier book, I therefore spoke of a psychoanalytic Exodus to the motherland that had already begun.[40] In a sense, this is no surprise. To put it in a feminist one-liner: half of humanity consists of women, the other half are their children.

Trauma

Ferenczi is now recognised as an absolute (but initially reviled) pioneer in psychoanalysis.[41] It seems as if Freud, in his analysis of the Oedipus myth, stops at the psyche of Oedipus, while Ferenczi also took into account that of Oedipus' parents, Laius and Jocasta. In this myth, they were the first to do 'evil.' Did they not leave him on Mount Cithaeron to be devoured by wolves? While Freud gradually shifted the emphasis from trauma to repression and/or the fantasy life, Ferenczi continued to emphasise its reality. He also included emotional intrusion and relational boundary violations in this. Regarding emotional parentification, he understood that children sacrifice their own emotional truth to maintain a connection with their caregivers. Especially when the latter are immature, emotionally needy, or abusive. His famous article on the confusion of tongues between adults and children provides an interpretative framework for this problem.[42] The child speaks the language of tenderness, and the adult speaks that of passion. The confusion arises because the child is drawn into the emotional or erotic power play of the adult. This does not even have to involve actual transgressive behaviour. More subtle emotional role reversals and unsymbolised questions or needs of adults are sufficient to disrupt the child's psyche.

The Wise Baby

The parentified child is subtly recruited to meet all kinds of adult needs: to comfort them, regulate their feelings, act as a confidant or a kind of partner. According to Ferenczi, the child becomes precocious but becomes internally fragmented and learns to trust only itself. In this context, he introduces the phenomenon of the 'wise baby': a child who shows remarkable insight, is very understanding and takes on a caring role.[43] However, this 'wisdom' is not a sign of optimal development but a defence against unbearable helplessness in an attempt to maintain attachment to the adult at all costs. We will see this again in Winnicott's False Self, but for Ferenczi, the cause lies explicitly in external trauma and not in the child's own imagination. The emotionally parentified child gives up spontaneity and authenticity, which can lead to deep dissociation of the person and later psychosomatic symptoms of all kinds. All this resonates with modern trauma theory and the childish prematurity described therein. He uses a striking and memorable metaphor for this. He compares the child to a piece of fruit damaged by a bird or an insect, which ripens (or rots) more quickly.[44] Intelligence takes a leap forward: an objective and emotionally detached, perceptive philosopher is formed within the child, as it were, who can observe from a distance and will intervene when all seems lost and hopeless. Ferenczi anticipates the concept of hypermentalisation or pseudomentalisation developed by Peter Fonagy and colleagues, who have conducted extensive research into the disturbed thought processes of borderline patients.[45] The child attempts to maintain itself in its insane environment by identifying with the adults. It becomes, as it were, a psychiatrist.[46] Harold Searles called this phenomenon 'the patient as therapist to the therapist.'[47] This refers to the hypervigilant and hypermentalising child who develops almost a sixth sense. In therapy, this translates into a patient who constantly 'scans' his therapist. It is therefore important that the analyst pays attention to excessive compliance or even submissiveness, which are remnants or derivatives of all this.

Identification with the Aggressor

Ferenczi also describes a mechanism that later became better known, through the work of Anna Freud, as 'identification with the aggressor.' In Ferenczi's work, however, the concept has a distinctly dissociative character. The child internalises the needs and perspectives of the adult in order to survive relationally, even when they threaten their own feelings, perceptions, or physical integrity. This inner and vertical split reflects what happens in emotional parentification. In fantasy and behaviour, the child takes on the position of the adult 'perpetrator' and suppresses (or even persecutes) their own dependence and vulnerabilities. For Ferenczi, this is not a neurotic defence mechanism but a survival strategy to avoid completely succumbing to overwhelm.[48] The net result of this is, for example, excessive feelings of guilt about one's own needs, chronic self-reproach, and confusion about boundaries and identity. A foreign object has been placed inside the person; the perpetrator has, as it were, been implanted in the child. The abused child attunes itself to the emotions and interests of the perpetrator and tries to identify with the aggressor by feeling their pain, tension, and passion, or by disqualifying the aggressor. The child no longer feels its own pain because it has killed itself: part of the person no longer exists. The aggressor is absorbed into the inner self in place of the dead part.

To be clear, Anna Freud's concept of identification with the aggressor was intended more as a neurotic defence mechanism. For her, it is a defence mechanism of the ego.[49] For example, the child feels threatened by punishment or aggression. To reduce fear, it identifies with the powerful aggressor and adopts their attributes (words, gestures, mannerisms). In this way, the child changes from a threatened object into an active, threatening figure. A passive-active reversal occurs, in which attack becomes the best form of defence.[50] This can be subtle (e.g., a child imitating the tone of voice of a teacher who reprimands them) or more serious (an abused child who later becomes violent towards others). However, Anna Freud continues to emphasise the ego defending itself against fear by identifying with the aggressor. As such, it is not a dissociative phenomenon, unlike in Ferenczi's trauma theory.

Ferenczi emphasises the passivity of the child who must do this in order to survive; Anna Freud emphasises the activity of the ego that does this to protect itself. In both senses, however, the concept remains crucial to the transgenerational transmission of intrapsychic and interpersonal patterns. Ferenczi is more relevant to the clinical treatment of abuse and violence, while Anna Freud's elaboration remains valuable for understanding everyday childhood defences and the role of identification in the formation of both the superego and character.

Ronald Fairbairn

A few years later, Ronald Fairbairn developed a very similar psychodynamic theory along these lines.[51] In his view, bad internal objects develop in all our lives. They refer to the internalised fantasy of an unresponsive parent. 'It is impossible to go through childhood without bad objects being internalised and repressed. These internalised bad objects are present in all of us in deeper regions.'[52] The introjection of and subsequent identification with bad objects is an adaptive mechanism whereby, according to Fairbairn, the child can regain control over a traumatising or neglectful dependency situation. 'Even if the child's parents are bad objects, the child cannot reject them… even if the child is rejected or neglected.'[53] The child would rather be 'bad' itself than have bad objects. By becoming bad, the child takes on the badness. It purifies its parents, washing them white, so to speak. This creates a new situation that is more bearable for the child: the parental objects are good and the child is bad. The child defends itself against bad objects by believing, 'I am bad; it is my fault.' The child defends the primary (love) object by taking on the parents' sins. Fairbairn calls this a 'moral defence' because if the child were good and the parents bad, this would be a disaster for the child. After all, the child would then be powerless. If, on the other hand, the child deserves the bad treatment, things can still turn out well. There is hope for redemption because the outside world is not bad. I quote the following statement verbatim because it plays such an important role in the psychodynamics of trauma: 'It is better to be a sinner in a world ruled by God than to live in a world ruled by the Devil.'[54] If the outside world is bad, the child cannot feel safe and cannot hope for redemption. There are only death and destruction, and therefore despair. Rather than that, the child would rather take on all the sins of Israel if necessary. In that context, I like to quote the following one-liner: Perfect parents exist, but they don't have children. In that sense, there are only two types of parents. Those who acknowledge their 'shortcomings'/'mistakes' and those who do not. In the latter case, the child is and always will be the one who pays the price.

Psychoanalytic Technique

Ferenczi was initially a hospital doctor and also worked with the sickest and most difficult (and often disadvantaged) patients.[55] This is an important reason why I often identify with him. In a Lacanian play on words, I believe he has mastered the art of '*le savoir/voir le* ça' and shows us the way for such psychopathology with his '*faire ainsi*.'[56] In conjunction with the views on trauma described above, Ferenczi did indeed revolutionise psychoanalytic technique, which is also relevant to the psychotherapy of parentification. He ventured into these technical innovations without being able to refer to theoretical reference points that were only developed later, such as Klein's projective identification, Bion's container-contained exchange, or Winnicott's transitional space.[57] However, they are all already implicitly contained in his clinical recommendations.

To begin with, Ferenczi was critical of the cold, neutral attitude of the analyst and sympathised with the need for empathic attunement, especially with traumatised patients. He gradually came to regard classic, rigid, and cold detachment as an expression of authority that is inherently traumatising for a patient (a fortiori if they were abused or parentified as a child).[58] A later leader of French institutional psychotherapy, Patrick Chemla, even speaks of *malicious* neutrality in connection with such a classically traditional psychoanalytic attitude in the treatment of so-called 'more serious' than purely neurotic psychopathology.[59]

In cases of emotional parentification, the child was deprived of appropriate emotional responsiveness and instead burdened with caring for the emotional lives of others. Psychotherapy should explicitly reverse this dynamic. Early relational trauma must be recognised, even when it is not manifestly abusive (at least according to the standards of outsiders). The patient must be allowed to regress in a completely safe environment and express needs that have remained unspoken until now. After all, the False Self must be stripped bare/deconstructed in order to establish or restore a connection with the True Self. According to him, psychoanalysis is primarily an interpersonal event in which transference and countertransference intertwine closely.

Ferenczi points out that the patient has often been analysed for much longer than his analyst. In that sense, the patient has more experience with psychoanalysis than his analyst. He will therefore defend the need for thorough and long-term analysis for the psychoanalyst. For Ferenczi, the best analyst is a patient who has cured himself. According to him, candidate analysts must first acknowledge their 'sick' sides in order to gain insight into their psychopathology and be cured of it. Only in this way can the analyst gain insight into his own limitations and blind spots.[60] In addition, he attaches great importance to honesty, transparency, flexibility, liveliness, humanity, repairing empathic ruptures, and the analyst's willingness to acknowledge his own limitations.

In particular, I will focus on the notion of 'tact' that he introduces and defines as the capacity for empathy.[61] It contributes to an 'elasticity of the analytical technique' that should be adapted to the patient's process rather than the other way around.[62] The analyst must, in his words, 'formally adopt the patient and allow him to share in the blessings of a normal nursery for the first time'[63] while caring for the patient. According to Ferenczi, the analyst becomes 'like a tender mother' to the patient.[64]

In contrast to Freud, who opposes *furor sanandi* as an obstacle, Ferenczi emphasises the importance of therapeutic ambition and generosity on the part of the therapist. He is willing to renounce an attitude of professional authority in order to dare to behave, together with the patient, like two anxious children who compare and share their experiences in order to get to know each other better. Such logic anticipates Antonino Ferro's idea that the patient is our best colleague.[65] In line with Lacan's '*la psychanalyse, c'est la science du particulier*' (psychoanalysis is the science of the particular), his psychoanalysis ultimately makes him a top scientist of *himself*!

Michael Balint: Primary Object Love and Basic Fault

Another Hungarian who thought along the same lines is Michael Balint. He introduced his concept of primary love[66] to refute Freud's concept of primary narcissism.[67] He thought that human beings are relationally oriented from the beginning. In this stage of primary object love, mother and child ideally live interdependently, with boundaries blurred, in a harmonious interpenetrating mix-up. He saw the origin of psychopathology in disruptions and failures of this experience. He developed a theory about the 'basic fault' that can occur when the child's dependency needs are not sufficiently met, resulting in damage to the child's psyche.

Balint distinguishes between a conflict model and a deficit model of psychopathology.[68] The latter occurs as a result of deficiencies in early childhood care and leads to a fault line, where early developmental needs were not met. Deep within the patient, this leads to feelings of emptiness, deadness, or meaninglessness. There is an insatiable longing for symbiotic fusion. Interpretation is not enough in this case. There is a need for a reparative emotional and relational experience. The patient may regress sufficiently. Balint spoke memorably of the analyst's stance at this stage: he must allow his patients to relate to him, or to exist with him, as if he were one of the primary substances. He should be like water that carries the swimmer or the earth that carries the walker. He must always be there, and he must be indestructible—as are water and earth. Dependence is thus supported by the psychotherapist's reliable and patient presence, which enables the 'wound' to heal through an empathetic approach.[69]

In parentification, the basic fault was covered up by a prematurely responsible and caring attitude, which paradoxically exacerbates the lack. The gap is widened, and it does not matter whether we describe this further in terms of Winnicott's False Self or in terms of Bion's reversal of the mother's alpha function. Here, too, both attachment and trauma theory provide further evidence. Disorganised attachment (often associated with abuse or neglect) causes role reversal.[70] Research on developmental trauma also shows that these children fluctuate between exaggerated responsibility and inner deadness.[71] Neurobiologically, chronic stress resonates with hippocampal regulation. The result is zero (rather than primary) process thinking, in which traumatic experiences are not symbolised and are stored as raw, undigested fragments.[72] Balint's idea of a kind of 'new beginning' takes centre stage. 'The new beginning helps the analysand to free himself of complex, rigid, and oppressive forms of relationship to his objects of love and hate … and to start simpler, less oppressive forms.'[73] Similar to Ferenczi, the analyst provides an environment in which dependence is not shameful and regression is sufficiently permitted so that a healing experience can unfold.

We will see that in British psychoanalysis, the Ferenczi line is followed not only by Balint but also by Donald Winnicott. According to André Green, the focus on the relational component of analysis, based on the mutual involvement between analyst and patient as equal—but in essence never symmetrical—actors, makes Ferenczi 'the father of modern psychoanalysis'[74] and Winnicott, in turn, 'the Ferenczi of the British Psychoanalytical Society.'[75]

Internal vs External Centre of Gravity

As has since become apparent, Sándor Ferenczi and Michael Balint were the first to theorise about the more maternal components that, in their view, should be included in the analytical work on 'early' disorders. In his clinical diary, Ferenczi refers to Goethe's *Faust*: 'Follow [the path] down to where the mothers live.'[76] Inspiration is the archaic mother-muse, from whom the *infant* must, in a sense, receive enough to be able to grow. This body of thought underlies the corrective-emotional[77] experience that is pursued in many later and supportive forms of psychotherapy.[78] Insofar as psychoanalysis remains essentially focused on discovering sometimes painful truths, it sometimes remains very sceptical of such a 'parental' approach. After all, a misapplication of these techniques could risk covering up or concealing this 'truth' under a cloak of love. However, clinical psychotherapeutic experience teaches us that this need not be the case at all.[79] Direct observations of children by René Spitz, Margaret Mahler, and Daniel Stern, for example, have amply confirmed the importance of such emotional and mental nourishment. John Bowlby initiated a whole series of large-scale studies on attachment, which were continued by Fonagy and his colleagues in a reciprocal intertwining with reflective functioning and mentalisation.[80] In another context, I have explained that all this belongs to the (Lacanian) register of the imaginary. It helps explain the relevance of the so-called non-specific therapeutic factors, which are effective across all (including non-psychoanalytic) psychotherapies.[81] I will return to all this in more detail later on.

In recent decades, there has also been a sharp rise in the popularity of so-called 'two-person psychology' within psychoanalysis. It replaces an individual and intrapsychic focus with an intersubjective and (socially) constructivist one. The psychoanalytic encounter is increasingly understood as a joint (ad)venture in which a shared psychological reality is fabricated by (the unconscious of) both partners. Because Klein and Winnicott take two extreme positions regarding this 'individual vs. context' controversy, I will first outline the framework from which they depart. After all, they represent the poles between which we must situate the clinic (in this case, of parentification).

Melanie Klein based her theory on intensive play therapy with (borderline) psychotic children who, despite their young age, were already seriously disturbed.[82] In this way, she reconstructed a hallucinatory and sadistic early childhood inner world. For Klein, the baby was highly differentiated from birth. According to her, the baby has imagination and an ego from the very beginning.[83] The inner world largely precedes the outer world, just as projection precedes introjection. What is internalised by the child is, for her, always and inevitably tainted by projection. For example, she believes that the first months of a child's life are dominated by the death drive[84] and by the fear of destruction and fragmentation that this causes. The baby defends itself against this by splitting off this destructive 'piece' and projecting it onto the object. She emphasises instinctual drives and the accompanying fantasy life at the expense of a relative neglect of the impact of the environment and external reality. Her technique focuses on an interpretative processing of transference and resistance (classical Freudian). She is notorious, for example, for her early and deep interpretations. Instead of focusing primarily on the patient, the patient is (according to critics) bombarded with interpretations in an overvaluation of words and interpretations.[85]

Donald Winnicott was not only an analyst but also worked for 40 years as a paediatrician with mothers and their babies. He developed his ideas partly from this paediatric practice with (more) normal mothers, their babies, and their mutual interactions. He paid a lot of attention to play and creativity, which he considered decisive signs of mental health. Based on this very different experience, he did not 'believe' in the constitutional nature of the death drive[86] but rather regarded aggression as a reactive product, namely as the result of disturbances or deficiencies in the environment.[87] For Winnicott, 'there is no such thing as a baby.' There is only an absolutely dependent being that can only survive by virtue of the 'primary maternal preoccupation'[88] of the nurturing mother. If the mother is (not perfect but) good enough, she provides the child with a 'continuity of being'[89] that can be regarded as an experience of fusion. The mother adapts almost completely to the child's needs. She offers gratification (e.g., the breast, warmth, support) wherever and whenever the child wants to create it (in a hallucinatory wish fulfilment). She also responds to her child's spontaneous gestures with good attunement ('mutuality').[90] In this way, the child is fed an illusion of imaginary omnipotence that allows it to experience divine/majestic moments and, to some extent, to be the creator of the world.

If the period of total dependence goes well enough, the child can develop a True Self from the core of its being and from its own centre of gravity. It can trust in a safe background figure and, in a state of non-integration,[91] surrender to peace and quiet in the presence of the mother.[92] For Winnicott, all these experiences are necessary (but insufficient) conditions for later creativity, relaxation, and enjoyment. However, if excessive disturbances occur during this initial period of absolute dependence, the baby feels threatened in its survival and experiences mortal fear. Only then does Winnicott's thinking come closer to Klein's negative and pathological-sounding views on hatred and sadism or on the schizoid-paranoid position. The child must, as it were, collaborate or mobilise all its forces to ward off the enemy (the external evil/ the 'bad' breast).

What often appears to the outside world and in hindsight as hatred and sadism is regarded by Winnicott as unintentional 'ruthlessness.'[93] It is the 'ruthlessness' that is the inevitable correlate of a life force that spares nothing and no one.[94] It is 'mouth-love'[95] in which devouring is still an integral part of love. In love, after all, the child only takes the feelings of the other into account in the later 'stage of concern,'[96] when it becomes aware of its dependence (previously misrecognised due to imaginary delusion). Concern and anxiety are its (positive and non-pathological) alternative terms for Klein's 'fears' from the depressive position.

For both Klein and Winnicott, the child only becomes aware of an inner evil in the second instance. It is only in a later phase that it becomes aware of the damage this evil has caused and can cause, and it is only from that moment on that it tries to make things right with the other person. Their very different concepts and use of language are based on a common idea, namely that the child only recognises the fact of its dependence after a prior period of omnipotent narcissism. They also attach great importance, in their own way, to the child who tries to (re)pair. In Klein's view, this (re)paration can be manic or depressive, depending on whether she starts from a schizoid-paranoid or a depressive position. In Winnicott's view, we also see how a False Self can develop in the first instance, in which any (personal) dependence is denied.

Holding and Interpretation: Not Either/or but Both/and

The theoretical contrast between the two should be strongly relativised in clinical practice. Winnicott's verbatim account of his own psychoanalytic work can convince anyone of the importance he attaches to holding and interpretation.[97] Conversely, Klein also attaches great importance to the quality of actual motherhood.[98]

Winnicott is important in every respect for understanding certain therapeutic imperatives regarding parentification. In the first years of life, the child is initially totally dependent on its environment and later relatively dependent. When psychopathology is rooted in these periods, Winnicott (like Ferenczi and Balint) considers deep regression to be therapeutically necessary in order to reconnect with the core of the True Self and to restart blocked ('*frozen*'[99]) development. This requires a holding environment[100] that can provide the necessary care and support while allowing the child in the patient to remain a child. In the case of the parentified patient, insight and mentalisation often appear insufficient. There is a strong tendency towards (in this case, therapeutically responsible) regression, in which the damage suffered must, as it were, be somewhat 'made up for.'

In fact, all patients who are (or need to be) treated in a residential setting need this kind of care and support. They need the safety, care, and protection that only a continuously available nursing role (the environmental mother) can offer them. In this context, we would like to point out that 'nursing' and 'nurturing,' as typical nursing terms, are identical to the terms used to describe the 'primary maternal preoccupation' with the baby. With all these problems, the patient (like the infant) needs us to accommodate certain illusions. For example, the illusion that the care provider has healing properties and knowledge is powerful, can offer protection, and can satisfy basic needs. An idealising transference arises, which we leave intact at first. We do not need to interpret it; we need to accept and respect it. The needy baby in the patient needs our more or less intensive care. He also needs mirroring, confirmation, support, and structure. By providing such a holding and facilitating environment, environmental deficits from the phase of absolute dependence can be (re)mediated. Narcissistic wounds can be repaired in a combined effort of (Fr.:) '*panser*' (anointing/connecting) and '*penser*' (thinking),[101] and support is a necessary but insufficient condition for psychotherapeutic work to begin. The process of change comes about in part because we allow the patient to use us.[102] Through interpretation, the entire transference-countertransference process is systematically provided with the necessary verbal footnotes.

Melanie Klein: Envy and Types of Reparation

As the founder of the object relations school of thought, Kleinian theory focuses on two particular areas. Firstly, it is primarily concerned with the primary objects that become part of our early childhood inner world, starting with partial objects (breast, penis) and later with the mother or father as whole objects. Fantasy is also central to her theory, specifically in its Kleinian sense, namely as a mental correlate of the drive.[103] In an initial (still animistic) phase, our earliest fears are related to (the image of) a gratifying/good or frustrating-persecuting/bad breast.[104] In the later depressive position, there is more of an image of the damaged parent who was damaged by the attacks in the previous phase and needs to be repaired. In parentification, this internal world is disrupted because the caregiver is failing in their role. The relationship is rather reversed, with the caregiver themselves in need and therefore dependent on the child to provide emotional support in various ways. The child experiences anxious concern about the fragility of the object and makes premature attempts to repair or rescue the parent. The reparative tendencies of the depressive position are precipitated before the child has been able to sufficiently integrate good and evil. This gives rise to excessive feelings of guilt, anxiety, and omnipotent (rescuer) fantasies. This lays the foundation for often lifelong difficulties with boundaries, chronic feelings of guilt or inadequacy, and, more generally, a hyper-empathic form of relating that ranges from strong antennae to the feeling of being an emotional sponge.

Apart from the observable interactions, much of this plays out invisibly through projective identification. Through this primitive defence mechanism, unbearable content is evacuated by the parent and the child has to metabolise it. The child must digest and process this unbearable content and somehow regulate it. It is, as it were, downloaded into the child, takes possession of the child's psyche, and must be mediated and remedied. The development of the child's own emotional life is hampered because the child's psyche has to organise itself around the parent's changing moods. Over time, the child's sense of self-worth even becomes dependent on the extent to which it can protect or stabilise the parent. This mindset becomes ingrained as a blueprint that shapes subsequent relationships between self and other. An unstable and distressed parent introjection and a responsible self form a template characterised by fear and guilt that repeatedly surfaces in the external and internal scenes.[105] Ultimately, this leads to a strict superego that does not allow the child to have its own needs, to compulsive caring for others, to difficulty in asking for or receiving help, and to an internal split between an omnipotent rescuer part and a helpless and abandoned part. Love must be earned, and any personal need or request is condemned as dangerous or selfish.

My compatriot Michel Thys also uses this Kleinian perspective to zoom in on the role that envy can play in parentification.[106] Envy is hatred towards and the desire to damage, spoil, and destroy a good object that is suspected, unlike the subject, of being omnipotent and having arbitrary power over the good it offers. Envy relates to the good object because it is good. The envious person cannot accept that they are not good themselves and that they must obtain goodness because they are not good themselves. In a nutshell: I can't stand having to get it![107]

Klein explicitly situates envy at the level of the relationship with one other object, which distinguishes it from jealousy. Jealousy is triangular and implies a rival third party: the other person has, takes, or threatens to take something good from me that I consider my own possession. I want the good thing back, but unlike in envy, I will not damage it. I want it back in good condition. In jealousy, I want the good thing (back); in envy, I want to be (like) the good thing.[108] Envy must also be distinguished from greed. Sucking the breast completely dry is about absorbing and devouring the good object. This is introjective identification: I become the object by absorbing it completely into myself. Envy, on the other hand, is a projective form of wanting to be the good object: I become the object by absorbing it completely (projective identification).

It should be clear that Klein's idea of envy closely aligns with Freud's idea of primary hatred of the object, the inability to tolerate (dependence on) the object as such. According to Freud, hatred is both older than and the parent of love.[109] It stems from the narcissistic ego's primordial rejection of stimuli from the outside world. Authors as diverse as Horacio Etchegoyen and Herbert Rosenfeld point to this connection between envy and narcissism.[110] Lacan also uses a neologism, *hainamoration* (a cocktail of love, hatred, and admiration), which is inextricably linked to the narcissistic-imaginary mirror stage: the sight of the whole arouses the hatred and envy of the fragmented/imagined.[111] Translated to the theme of parentification: parents are big children and children are little parents. Parents want to be children (again) and children want to be parents (already).

Envy is the projective and violent intrusion into the object in order to be the object itself and thus to abolish its objecthood. In overconfident desperation, I promote myself to breast! The child wants to be the parent itself. We might perhaps speak here of envious parentification.[112] Any experience of dependence, let alone helplessness, is extremely threatening to the child and must be covered up by the illusion of triumphant self-empowerment. It presents itself as invulnerable, headstrong, precocious, and unapproachable. The envious parentified adult remains on guard and does not really allow others in, distrusts or despises what others have to offer, and does everything on their own. They are a well-filled and self-satisfied breast. Kleinian thinking allows us to describe two other subtypes of parentification: obsessive or penitent parentification and manic or triumphant parentification. In clinical reality, of course, they always occur in combination. Penitent parentification involves a combination of grief and remorse: the child mourns the damage/destruction of the object and feels remorse because it assumes that this loss is the result of its own envy. After envy comes regret. The baby who has harmed its mother by biting and tearing her develops fantasies in which it puts the pieces back together and repairs her.[113] In extremis, the fear of the death of the beloved will trigger a very strong, irresistible urge to repair.[114] Manic or triumphant parentification is a kind of intermediate or transitional form between envy and repentance. In manic parentification, there is also a tendency to repair, but this easily turns into an almighty feeling of triumph because it is mainly aimed at undoing the unbearable dependence. The repair starts out 'benign,' as it were, but quickly sinks into the psychological quagmire of envy and narcissism. The depressive tendency to repair is present, but it is too weak and cannot compete with the suction force of paranoid envy. While obsessive penitential parentification is a self-sacrificing, dependent form of parentification, manic parentification is a triumphant, condescending form.

Donald Winnicott: Holding and True Self

Emotional parentification is a relational aberration in which the child is explicitly or implicitly enlisted to regulate the parent's emotional life. This may involve comforting or encouraging a depressed parent, mediating in conflicts, being used as a confidant or confidante, or as a stand-in for a partner who is absent or gives up on the relationship. The core of Winnicott's thinking naturally revolves around a mother who is good enough to adapt to the child without overwhelming or abandoning them. Such a mother is not perfect, but she nevertheless creates a sufficiently solid and consistent environment in which early childhood experiences of omnipotence, spontaneity, and disintegration can unfold in a safe manner. This holding is reversed in parentification. It is the child who must provide holding to an emotionally unstable, immature or narcissistically wounded parent and act as a container for their emotions.

The True Self goes into hiding or becomes dissociated. In its place, the False Self emerges as a defensive structure to meet the parent's needs and desires at the expense of authentic expression of one's own needs and desires. The False Self is 'compliant and aims at preserving relationships even if it must sacrifice the self.'[115]

Of course, this is not deliberate deception, but rather an almost visceral strategy of psychological survival for the sake of relational continuity. The parentified child is mature, obliging, helpful, and emotionally sensible, but over time suffers from depression, emptiness, and loss. In healthy development, the significant Other is calm enough for the child to gradually come into contact with their own inner self. In parentification, on the other hand, the child is overwhelmed by parental needs, confessions, or emotional fragility. These disrupt optimal integration and lead to hyper-adaptive behaviour in which the person concerned constantly effaces themselves in relationships, takes on excessive responsibility, and experiences feelings of guilt, and finds it difficult to express their own needs or interests (or have them represented). Entirely in line with Ferenczi, psychotherapy should create a space where spontaneity can emerge, where the False Self can be understood and recognised as an attempt to survive, where regression can take place to allow the True Self to blossom, and where missed opportunities for emotional care can be mourned. The False Self is not actively attacked, but conditions are created in which the True Self can thrive. In other words, Winnicott is less concerned with interpretation (as Klein is) than with realising an experience. The patient must (re)learn what it means to be held, to play, to simply be allowed to be there instead of having to do all kinds of things. The varying combination of holding and interpretation that we see in Klein and Winnicott is extended in the difference in technique between Otto Kernberg (with psychoanalytic psychotherapy that focuses on analysis of [negative] transference) and

Heinz Kohut (where a tailored combination of empathic mirroring and optimal frustration ensures the creation of a cohesive Self).

Wilfred Bion: Container-Contained, Attacks on Linking

But first, let us consider Wilfred Bion, who provides highly relevant and profound concepts for understanding the invisible (and often infraverbal) emotional burden inherent in parentification. The core of his approach is how thoughts and emotional experiences only take shape in the presence of a caregiver who metabolises raw mental states. With a nod to Descartes: she (the [m]other) thinks, therefore I am. If and only if I am thought of as *Homo sapiens* and *sentiens* can I develop as such. In emotional parentification, this 'container-contained'[116] relationship is completely reversed. The result: premature (pseudo)maturity and, in the long term, a detrimental combination of hypermentalisation (of another person's state of mind) and hypomentalisation (of one's own state of mind).

Bion introduced the now-popular concept of containment: the caregiver's ability to engage in reverie—that is, to receive, hold, and digest the child's raw emotional experiences (in his terminology, beta elements). Through the mother's intuitive presence, chaos is transformed into cosmos and returned to the child in a more digestible form. In this way, the child (also) develops alpha function, defined as the ability to think and symbolise and thus to tolerate and endure emotions.[117] In emotional parentification, the child is prematurely 'promoted' to a proto-container. Prematurely, because it does not yet have a sufficiently developed psychological 'apparatus' and therefore becomes overloaded. Bion also expanded Klein's originally purely fantastical concept of projective identification into a communicative mechanism.[118] The caregiver evacuates or downloads mental contents into the child, who is forced to embody this part and organise themselves around it. The child's psyche is, as it were, colonised by an affect that is foreign to it, with which it nevertheless identifies. It becomes, as it were, a psychological appendix (or appendicitis!) of the parent who hides their own subjective truth from everyone.

One of Bion's most original contributions is his concept of 'attacks on linking.'[119] This is a defence mechanism that arises when emotional experiences become too overwhelming. The parentified child is often exposed to contradictions, emotional chaos, or a loss of boundaries. For example, the parent may be dependent on their child and, at the same time, hate, idealise, and use them. The child cannot process such mixed messages and defensively switches off their own thinking ability. Instead of connecting, they disconnect. For example, they break the connection between feeling and meaning, between inside and outside, between self and other. What cannot be thought is expelled or split off.

Later, this can 'take its toll' in various ways, such as alexithymia (the inability to read one's own mental content), inhibited thinking or excessive intellectualisation, and/or psychosomatic symptomatology. The child functions well in critical/precarious situations but is unable to reflect or symbolise properly. In emotional parentification, the caregiver is unavailable or intrusive, and the child is not allowed *to feel* good but must *function* well. Inadequate containment leads to evacuation rather than integration. Unmentalised affects become permanently embedded in the child's body or behaviour but cannot be thought. Over time, this leads to an impoverished inner world, limited emotional language, hyperreactivity without understanding, emotional numbness, or burnout.

Such psychodynamic and psychogenetic mechanisms naturally imply a therapeutic logic. The psychotherapist's most important task is to receive the beta elements, absorb them without retaliation or fragmentation, and return them in symbolised form. In other words, Bion focuses on the emotional architecture of thought itself. The therapist fulfils a musical function, providing symbolic forms with which the patient can forge his fragmented experiences into a more comprehensible whole. While Klein mainly talked about the internalisation of harmful or damaged objects and Winnicott about the False Self and developmental interferences, Bion zooms in on undigested emotions, projective identifications, and dissolving forces. Psychotherapy restores the ability to think under emotional pressure.[120]

Otto Kernberg vs Heinz Kohut: Internal vs External Focus Once Again

For completeness, here are two more recent authors who further elaborate on the aforementioned inspirations. Parentification is never explicitly mentioned by Otto Kernberg, but it is implicitly woven into his theories on object relations, personality development, and 'early' psychopathologies such as narcissistic and borderline organisation. From an integration of the ego-psychological and Kleinian perspectives, he describes how the development of an integrated self depends on the internalisation of consistent, affectively charged self- and object-representations in early childhood. Parentification disrupts this development. I quote: 'The child's early identifications with powerful or helpless figures may interfere with the integration of self-representations, resulting in identity diffusion.'[121] For him, this identity disorder is one of the essential characteristics of borderline organisation. Instead of an integrated image of self and other, an internal world emerges characterised by splitting: the parent is alternately idealised and devalued, perceived as needy and demanding, weak and domineering.[122] This is also typical of parentification, in which the child feels both responsible and overwhelmed. In addition, a primitive and often sadistic superego develops that is more persecutory than protective.[123]

When the child is used to reinforce the parent's sense of self, Kernberg refers to this as narcissistic transference: the parent projects his or her fantasies of grandeur or need for mirroring onto the child.[124] Such children may later develop aspects of pathological narcissism themselves, in which the self and self-esteem remain fragile and dependent on ever-changing life circumstances and environmental factors. This mainly concerns what is referred to as vulnerable or 'thin-skinned narcissism.'[125] In the transference-focused psychotherapy developed by Kernberg and his colleagues, the parentified patient can place the therapist in the position of a helpless object that needs care and understanding. These transference distortions must, of course, be interpreted.[126]

It is also appropriate here to refer to the thinking of Heinz Kohut, who developed his own self psychology. Like Winnicott, he emphasises the positive aspects of narcissism in relation to creativity, humour, and wisdom. For him, psychological growth results from two contrasting processes: empathic mirroring and optimal frustration. His therapeutic technique is largely based on empathy. For him, pathology corresponds to the deficit model and is the result of empathic deficits and/or traumatic disruption of the mother-child dyad, resulting in 'nameless preverbal aggression.'[127] Although Kohut, like Kernberg, does not explicitly mention parentification, his views on the self-object, the development of a cohesive self, and narcissistic dependence/vulnerability provide fruitful inspiration in this regard. From a Kohutian perspective, parentification can be the result of trauma or poor attunement, whereby the child has to function as the parent's self-object instead of being able to satisfy its own narcissistic needs with this parent. The child does not exist as a separate subject but plays a key role in the parent's narcissistic economy.[128] The child needs mirroring to confirm joy, initiative, or other emotions. They must be able to look up to the parent as a source of calmness and strength that can be relied upon, and they seek recognition, similarity, and connection in the other person. These are all necessary to create a cohesive sense of self that forms the basis for sufficient self-confidence, ambition, and emotional regulation. Emotional parentification often involves a chronic lack of empathy, experienced, so to speak, 365 days a year. This results in narcissistic vulnerability in varying combinations with excessive empathy for others, shame about one's own needs or limitations, a fragmented self-image in the face of conflict or failure, and difficulty dealing with disappointment or criticism. As with Winnicott, the therapeutic emphasis is on a corrective emotional experience in which the patient can still experience how it feels to be received, affirmed, and appreciated in the mind and heart of the therapist. Often, for the first time, the patient experiences not being *needed* by the therapist. Their feelings lead to attunement and are no longer rejected. Feelings of dependence are not shameful, and emotional reactions are mirrored and truly taken to heart.

John Bowlby: Attachment and Compulsive Caregiving

John Bowlby described how children who are confronted with parental rejection or loss develop defensive strategies to maintain the attachment bond.[129] When the parent fails as a source of security, the child attempts to emotionally stabilise the parent through 'compulsive caregiving' (a form of over-adaptation and over-responsibility).[130] On the other hand, his student Mary Ainsworth observed in her 'strange situation' study that some children (especially those with an ambivalent/resistant attachment style) constantly try to reassure others and regulate their emotional state. This behaviour reflects the internalisation of an insecure working hypothesis: 'My parent needs me to feel good.' The child learns to suppress their own needs in favour of relational stability, a dynamic that can lead to excessive empathy, perfectionism, and difficulties with dependence in adulthood.[131] From a Bowlbian perspective, parentification can therefore be seen as a defensive attachment strategy: an attempt to maintain closeness by providing care rather than receiving it. This reversal of care undermines the development of a secure Internal Working Model in which the self can feel dependent without fear of rejection.[132] The clinical echoes of this are visible in adult relationships in which care and love are confused with control, and in which affective boundaries become blurred.

We can simply distinguish the different attachment styles on the basis of two axes (anxiety and avoidance) in four quadrants:[133] 1) secure: characterised by low avoidance and low anxiety; 2) preoccupied: characterised by high anxiety and low avoidance; 3) dismissive-avoidant: characterised by low anxiety and high avoidance; and 4) anxious-avoidant. The latter corresponds to a 'disorganised attachment style.'[134] The first three attachment styles are basically adaptive. None of the three necessarily indicates a deviation or pathology. After all, this is an ecological system. In times of poverty, stress, war, and migration, an avoidant attachment style increases the likelihood of survival, even at the expense of emotional security. A preoccupied attachment style is the most appropriate solution for an inconsistent family. By clinging, the child increases the parent's proximity and predictability. Secure attachment is best suited to a normal, loving, and sensitive family. There is a strong correlation between parents' reflective function and children's later attachment style. This is mediated by parents' mentalising ability.[135] Secure attachment is associated with greater tolerance of stress, better resilience to later stressors, and better memory function. A parent who, based on their own needs, places excessive demands on the child's attachment system also hinders the development of proximal systems, such as exploration and play.

An avoidant attachment style can result from parentification. It may be best for the child to keep the parent/other person at a safe distance to safeguard their own development! The person concerned becomes a headstrong do-it-yourselfer and may later have difficulty with the emotional closeness required for intimate relationships. However, I will mainly discuss preoccupied and disorganised attachment styles because they are most closely correlated with emotional parentification. The preoccupied or 'resistant' attachment style is characterised by inconsolability and rejection of the parent. These children do cling but cannot be reassured by the parent's presence. They are therefore unable to use the parent figure as a safe haven. They express their feelings of anger or despair in the event of separation.[136] In adults, this attachment style is called ambivalent-preoccupied, also known as overly involved or 'entangled.' In the 'Adult Attachment Interview,' the story of such preoccupied adults is usually too long.[137] They are angry, passive, or overwhelmed by unpleasant experiences and often somewhat confused. The self and others are also confused about grammatical subject forms. The sense of self-identity seems weak. The same applies to the distinction between the present and the past. They often use jargon ('my mother was borderline') or childish language and are unable to express their experiences well in words. The reflective function is low. According to infant research, interactive regulation appears to overwhelm self-regulation in this group.[138] This is noticeable in interactions between mothers and their young children when the mother fails to notice the baby's signals of wanting to withdraw (as an attempt at self-regulation) and continues to seek contact. Children who were not given sufficient space for self-regulation in their first year of life were found to have a 'resistant' attachment style at thirteen months.[139] Too little attunement is not good, but neither is too much. Children who were vocally and expressively 'in tune' with their mothers for 50% of the interaction time were later found to be securely attached; it is therefore really about being good enough, not about being perfect.

In terms of the later (and subsequently discussed) mentalisation theory, it is assumed that parents with preoccupied children did not mark the affects they mirrored. The difference between the child's affect or emotion and that of the parent is not sufficiently emphasised, as a result of which the child does not feel seen as the 'owner' of a feeling that is not yet bearable. It seems as if mother and child are living in the same hurricane of feelings. Later on, the child does not see itself in the parent's eyes, but sees a (love) hungry or disappointed child in the parent. In a normal population, preoccupied attachment is found in 15% of cases. In a clinical population, it is found three times more often.[140]

Parentification can also be a reaction to disorganised attachment. The term was first introduced by Mary Main and her colleagues, who, while video-recording babies in their Bay Area study, found a small group that exhibited strange behaviour at certain moments. They suggested that this disorganised attachment would occur in children whose parents were simultaneously a source of security and fear. This hypothesis has since been amply confirmed empirically.[141] Of the abused toddlers studied by Dante Cicchetti and colleagues, 80% were disorganisedly attached.[142] According to Karlen Lyons-Ruth, affective communication with the child is disrupted.[143] As a result, the child cannot develop a consistent representation of the world's predictability and remains insecure, prey to changing, inconsistent implicit images of self and others (just like the mother herself). The child, therefore, remains anxious and avoidant. Longitudinal studies show that such disruption of mother-child interactions plays an important role in the later development of post-traumatic symptoms. Disorganisation appears to play a particular role in 'numbing' and avoidance.[144]

In preoccupied attachment, the behaviour of the parentified child serves to make the parent as predictable as possible. Disorganisation of attachment is something else entirely. It primarily concerns the level of mental representations of self and others, rather than behaviour. The latter can even be particularly rigid, coercive, and controlling. In contrast to organised attachment styles, disorganised attachment means a breakdown of strategies for regulating closeness and security. Disorganisation leads to dysregulation of emotions, stress, and autobiographical memory. Representations of self and others are confused and confusing. The child is not a clear 'owner' of feelings and thoughts, there is no coherent sense of identity, and reflecting on one's own feelings and thoughts evokes anxiety: the reflective function is not strong. The assumption is that the world is hostile and unpredictable, with disasters constantly lurking.

According to the Dutch Trimbos Institute, there are 1.6 million children under the age of twenty-two in the Netherlands with one or both parents diagnosed with a mental disorder.[145] Parentified children with mentally ill parents experience their parents as both helpless and dangerous. The danger comes from outside and from within. After all, they also experience themselves, with their normal emotions and needs, as monstrous creatures who are dangerous to others. Every emotion can destroy the weak and pitiful mother.

I will give a brief clinical vignette.[146] Helen has a mother with a dissociative disorder. From the age of six, she took care of her mother. She knows her mother's different personalities and addresses them accordingly. She put her mother to bed, woke her up, and stood next to the kitchen sink watching as her mother prepared food. She did not ask for care for herself and taught herself not to need anything. When she went to school and was bullied, she hid this from her mother. She taught herself not to become attached to anyone, she says. 'Then it hurt less.' From the age of thirteen, she managed her mother's financial affairs. When Helen comes to therapy, because she is so gloomy she can hardly put into words what she is experiencing inside. Every feeling is a sign of weakness that must be kept under control at all costs. The psychotherapist remains a distant stranger to her, who, in her perception, wants to 'transform' her: something she resists tooth and nail. A question about her feelings is experienced as an unauthorised intrusion. Only much later is she able to express that she experiences every word, every action of another person as dangerous, an attack on her and her precarious sense of self-esteem. Keeping everything at arm's length goes so far that she has no contact with others. She also does not dare to think about what she herself feels. Not least, Helen's treatment will need to focus on learning to tolerate her own emotions and thoughts so that she can recognise them as *her own*.[147]

Peter Fonagy: Mentalisation and the Alien Self

Peter Fonagy is undoubtedly one of the most influential psychoanalysts and developmental psychologists of recent decades. He developed his own unique lens (consisting of mentalisation, attachment, and epistemic trust) through which the psychodynamics of parentification can be further explained from a new and illuminating perspective. Emotional parentification essentially involves a failure of mentalisation on the part of the parent. This disrupts the development of self-awareness, affect regulation, and interpersonal trust. Fonagy defines mentalisation as the ability to understand oneself and others as persons with thoughts, feelings, and intentions. Children are not born with these abilities but develop them through a secure and attuned attachment relationship.

In emotional parentification, the parent falls short and/or the roles are reversed. The child has to understand and deal with the parental feelings. It prematurely develops a pseudo- or hyper-mentalising ability, reading the other person. It regulates (pseudo-maturely) the parent's emotions, becomes a source of support and comfort (role reversal), or becomes a confidant or surrogate partner (enmeshment). This leads to disorganised attachment, in which the child feels both responsible for and threatened by the parent's inner world.

In his latest publications, Fonagy puts forward the concept of 'epistemic trust.' Can the child trust that the other person's communication is relevant, meaningful, and benevolent?[148] If not, epistemic hypervigilance develops. The child scans the other person's mood and expectations but rejects or is sceptical of what the other person says about their own state of mind or motives. Emotional distance or compulsive caring has other consequences: they have difficulty with positive affirmation, distrust parental figures or authorities, or they become self-made or 'bad pupils.' Their 'empathy' serves mainly defensive purposes. They quickly sense the atmosphere and feel what is or is not expected, while they lack or lose touch with themselves. In other words, their empathy is instrumental. It serves more to avoid conflict or abandonment than to foster genuine connection.

For optimal development, the caregiver must mirror the child's inner world in a marked and attuned/contingent manner.[149] Parents do this involuntarily, for example, by widening their eyes or raising their voice. Through their facial expressions, melody, prosody, and rhythm, they indicate that they understand the child's feelings but do not feel the same way. When such mirroring is lacking, a False Self can develop, according to Winnicott. Fonagy adds to this with what he calls the 'Alien Self': a phenomenon that occurs more in borderline than in narcissistic problems. Unmarked emotions are experienced as contagious, overwhelming, or downright dangerous. An indigestible and inexpressible Alien Self is expelled through projective identification and ends up in the child, damaging its developing mentalising capacity. When you are repeatedly misunderstood and (due to parental transference, projection, or projective identification) are constantly attributed the same 'strange' mental contents or intentions, you inevitably become more or less confused about yourself.

As always, the psychodynamic and psychogenetic processes described above provide *direct* inspiration for psychotherapy.[150] After all, the Internal Working Models (and the caregiving behaviour based on them) of the parents are passed on to their offspring with their mother's milk/spoonful.[151] This fateful logic is significantly tempered by psychotherapy aimed at the parents, which increases their sensitivity and reflective functioning.[152] It should create a space where the self can be mentalised without any demand for reciprocity, without risk of abandonment, and without the parentified person having to bear any responsibility for the other. In this way, epistemic trust can gradually be rebuilt. The other person is safe, responsive, and reliable. The patient can thus learn to differentiate between their own needs, feelings, and intentions and those of others: a necessary (but of course insufficient) condition for a more authentic life and experience.

Infant Research: It Takes Two to Tango

As has now become apparent, parentification is often described as a child bearing too much responsibility in a dysfunctional family. The classic image is that of a child who matures too early and who cares for, mediates, comforts, soothes, and organises. However, infant research shows that the seeds of this can already be seen in the first micro-interactions between baby and parent. These earliest relational patterns form a *ground script* in which self-awareness, emotional regulation, and later relational expectations are embedded. The work of Margaret Mahler, Beatrice Beebe, Daniel Stern, Edward Tronick, and Allan Schore offers a developmental matrix for rethinking parentification as a lack of co-regulation and a reversal of affective functions from the first year of life.

Margaret Mahler described the birth of the psychic self as a process of increasing differentiation and separation from the symbiosis with the mother.[153] Crucial to this is that the young parent can carry what the child cannot yet regulate in these early stages. But when the mother is psychologically unstable, needy, or emotionally unavailable, a subtle reversal occurs. Instead of being able to unfold in the practising phase and find support in the rapprochement phase, the child emotionally bends back towards the parent. The early illusion of autonomy (Mahler observed toddlers crawling around with a sense of omnipotence) can become a pseudo-autonomy in such a context. The apparent independence actually becomes a primitive caregiving task: the child develops behaviour to stabilise the parent's emotional state. This stunts separation-individuation, and the self is not given the space to experience itself as a source of impulses, desires, and boundaries. The development of subjectivity is exchanged for relational monitoring.

Beatrice Beebe's microanalyses show how fundamental 'dyadic synchrony' is to the development of affect regulation.[154] In healthy interactions, mismatch and repair alternate: it is not the failure of attunement that causes harm, but the absence of repair. Chronic misattunement places an unbearable burden on the baby: instead of a parent who repairs, it is the baby who keeps trying to connect. Beebe describes how infants develop a pattern in which their own affective responses narrow in favour of the relationship.

Original spontaneity gives way to relational control. This creates a form of proto-parentification: the baby's body and face become instruments for regulating the other. In adulthood, this often leads people to feel others' emotions more quickly than their own and to confuse security with harmony at any price.

Daniel Stern described early development as a gradual construction of different 'senses of self' (emergent, core, subjective, and verbal), of which the subjective self is a milestone: the moment when the child experiences that its inner world is recognised by another.[155] However, when the parent relies on the child for emotional continuity, the result is not *a self-with-other*, but a *self-for-other*. The intersubjective space becomes instrumental. Instead of getting to know itself through mirroring, the child mainly learns what the other needs it to be. This is the psychological core of parentification: the other becomes not a partner in subjectification, but a client.

Tronick's Still-Face Experiment shows the essence: the baby tries to revive the unresponsive parents: smiling, making sounds, stretching out its arms. It searches, reaches out, recovers, and when the other person does not participate, its physiological and affective system collapses and we see sadness or freezing.[156] In families where emotional unavailability, depression, trauma, or dissociation are present, this one-off experiment becomes a rule of life. The child internalises the task: keep reviving the other person. Tronick describes how consciousness can only expand within co-regulation.[157] In this light, parentification is a collapse of the dyadic space in which the child alone structurally bears the burden of recovery.

Allan Schore demonstrates that affect regulation and attachment are anchored in right-hemispheric networks established in the first eighteen months.[158] This means that a baby who structurally regulates the parent develops a pattern of hypervigilance and focus on the other person, not only psychologically but also neurobiologically. The stress system becomes programmed for vigilance and relationship maintenance rather than exploration and spontaneous self-expression. As a result, the later adult parentified patient often remains relationally 'on': scanning, anticipating, avoiding conflict, and afraid of emotional rejection. The roots lie not in character, but in biography—and, more precisely, in the first biographical layer of the body.

Infant research has also made it clear that parentification must be distinguished from other phenomena. For example, there is precocious maturity: the child is intellectually advanced but not emotionally burdened. There is also such a thing as high sensitivity: the child has heightened perception but lacks a care-taking script. Finally, there are also normal empathic care tendencies, but these are transient and situational. Parentification occurs when regulation is reversed, linked to relational responsibility, and associated with a conditional sense of self: 'I am allowed to exist as long as I care for others.' Clinically, this is reflected in transference as cautious, harmonising, self-effacing tendencies and a deep sense of shame about one's own needs. Therapy here requires not so much a technique as a certain attitude. If the earliest task was 'I must regulate the other,' then the new experience must be 'I am allowed to receive without caring.' Based on infant research, this presupposes three core psychotherapeutic tasks: continuous regulation of the affective climate; giving language to desires, anger, shame, or neediness; and tolerating conflicts, breaks, and silences without breaking the connection.

Neuropsychoanalysis: A Conversation of Bodies

Thanks in particular to the work of Allan Schore, neuropsychoanalytic insights and findings are relevant not only to relational, non-specific, or generic factors in psychoanalytic psychotherapy, but also to the parentified patient. Early relational trauma disrupts the maturation of the right hemisphere, which impedes the ability to form attachments and process emotions.[159] Emotional parentification indeed implies a biopsychosocial interplay: early care requirements leave their mark on neural circuits (e.g., on the HPA axis or on empathic networks) and they luxate defence mechanisms. All this has long-term consequences for the adult's emotional health, identity, and relationships.[160] After all, the development of our brains is strongly influenced by our earliest relationships. The prefrontal cortex, which is responsible for decision-making and impulse control, continues to develop throughout childhood. Chronic activation of the HPA axis increases cortisol levels, which has a detrimental effect on both the prefrontal cortex and the hippocampus (memory, stress regulation). Hyperactivity of the amygdala leads to increased emotional reactivity (anxiety, hypervigilance). Excessive development of mirror neurons (which play a key role in empathy) leads to increased attunement to others' emotions, but also to burnout and boundary blurring (enmeshment). Changes in the brain's default mode shift the focus to the other person and at the same time neglect what relates to the self. Hypermentalisation of other people's emotions, accompanied by alexithymia of one's own emotional world, correlates with reduced connectivity in the anterior cingulate cortex and the insula, areas crucial for emotional awareness. Prolonged stress can cause epigenetic changes (e.g., methylation of stress-related genes), resulting in increased susceptibility to anxiety and depression.[161]

Twenty-five years of interdisciplinary research characterised by an integration of neuroscience, developmental psychology, attachment theory, and psychoanalysis resulted in what Schore calls his 'right-brain psychotherapy.' In his view, it forms the basis and breeding ground for the verbal talking cure, which is more likely to originate in the left hemisphere. This involves dyadic, intensely emotional, and neurobiologically determined processes in mutual right-hemispheric communication; 'a listening and feeling cure.'[162] This 'right brain turn' runs parallel to developments in neuroscience (Jaak Panksepp, Antonio Damasio), infant research (Daniel Stern, Edward Tronick), and the 'relational turn' within psychoanalysis (Stephen Mitchell, Jessica Benjamin),[163] all of which place non-verbal communication at the forefront as the most important vehicle for change.

The right hemisphere develops earlier than the left and is by far the most important during our first thousand days: the period in which our sense of self, attachment patterns, and affect regulation are established.[164] It regulates autonomous arousal and stress responses; processes primary emotions and physical sensations; recognises facial expressions, tone, and prosody; contains non-verbal and implicit memory systems; and houses the core self through changing circumstances. For Schore, it is therefore the biological substrate of the unconscious. It mediates affective meaning as well as the resonance between I and you, self and other. The left hemisphere only translates and symbolises all this in the second instance. However, part of the emotional truth is lost in translation. I paraphrase: 'The right brain is the seat of the implicit self: the bodily-based self that psychotherapy seeks to reach and heal.'[165]

Building on Bowlby, Ainsworth and Tronick, Schore describes the earliest mother-child dyad as the original matrix for psychobiological regulation.

The mutual right-hemispheric attunement through gaze, facial expression, tone and rhythm modulates the child's arousal and mood and lays the foundation for both secure attachment and self-regulation. It determines the right-hemispheric 'architecture.'[166] This essentially involves a conversation between bodies, a kind of dance between mother and child that 'precedes and exceeds language.' It is therefore nothing less than the stuff that (early) transference and countertransference are made of.

This has important therapeutic implications for the so-called non-specific therapeutic factors. Safety is more important than insight. The patient must feel emotionally supported/cared for. Presence is more important than intervention/interpretation because right-hemispheric synchrony is a necessary condition for verbal meaning. Attunement is more important than neutrality and, finally, recovery is more important than perfection. Disruptions in the connection are inevitable but repairing them is necessary for emotional growth. Psychotherapy must be guided by an ethic of presence and compassion. At the deepest level, he even calls psychotherapy 'an act of love…'[167]

Jacques Lacan: Signifier and Lack, Mirror and Phallus

After this long exodus to the pre-Oedipal motherland, we return to the fatherland with Jacques Lacan. We will see that his rationalist approach takes precedence over the empirical. We also immediately move from the imaginary to the symbolic register and from the order of need to that of desire. This latter distinction is a key point for Lacan and, in a sense, forms the basis of his theory of subjectivity, the unconscious and psychoanalytic practice. Before zooming in on a Lacanian psychoanalysis of parentification, some introductory context is necessary to avoid unnecessary 'confusion of tongues' (with a nod to Ferenczi).

As with all mammals, the mother-child relationship forms the extrauterine matrix for our further development. But is it really just a matter of 'need' for human children? Authors such as Bowlby, Ainsworth, and Fonagy consider secure attachment to be a neurobiological and evolutionary system aimed at survival. The child seeks proximity to the caregiver in situations such as fear, pain, or fatigue. This seems as universal and vital as food or oxygen. Lacan changes this logic because the Big Other is not only a 'person' but also a symbolic field (the discourse of micro- and macro-culture). In other words, just like the child, we willingly or unwillingly enter the realm of law and language. The Big Other speaks, asks, demands: 'Sleep!' 'Say thank you,' 'Behave properly.' Every social and symbolic context is full of questions that interpellate the subject. For the child, the mother (as the first representative of the Other) is indeed the one who provides answers, but she is also the one who makes (implicit or explicit) demands. The Other's question is therefore always ambiguous: it is supposedly about satisfying a need (e.g., eat everything on your plate), but there is always an aspect of personal desire (if not need) hidden within it (e.g., I expect you to like this). What the Big Other (exactly) desires is both mysterious and frightening—especially because it can never be fully translated. Here, the spectre of the Big Other appears, consuming me, using me, or reducing me to a mere passive object/suffering object.

The *need/requirement/besoin* refers to our survival or the natural needs of the body. In principle, it can be satisfied by an adequate object (food, drink, sleep, etc.), but Lacan emphasises that this dimension is not sufficient to speak of human life. As soon as the need is expressed in language (starting with the crying baby), a shift occurs from the biological to the psychological register. The child asks not only for milk, but also for love, recognition, and presence. Lacan therefore argues that in every *question/demande* there is a residue that cannot be reduced to the satisfaction of the need.[168] Desire is the name for this residue: the supposed surplus that arises when the need is expressed in language. Desire is caused by a missing object. It is the *manque-à-objet* that Lacan will eventually call the object small a (or *objet-cause* as the 'object' that *causes* desire).

The question is a need expressed in language. It is directed at another and is therefore essentially intersubjective.[169] It is the other who responds to what is read as a question. The child is thus incorporated into a meaningful universe with the (mirror of the) little other-equal who also embodies the Big Other (and its micro- and macro-culture of language and signifiers). For Lacan, from his first seminar onwards, the question is essentially a 'question about *love.*'[170] This question may conceal a need, but its answer is primarily symbolic. The child is inevitably confronted with an Other who cannot (entirely) satisfy its needs. The child tries to adapt by being what the Other lacks, but in turn fails fatally. This law introduces the lack that 'causes' or gives rise to desire.

Freud already stated that the drive is never fully satisfied and continues to revolve around a kind of 'urge.'[171] Lacan radicalises this by stating that desire is structurally unfulfillable. It is the residue that arises from the symbolic mediation of the question. This desire is also always the desire of the Other (objective and subjective genitive). We desire not only *what* the Other desires, but also *that* the Big Other recognises our desire and confirms our object of desire. A Lacanian understanding of psychoanalysis is not merely about satisfying needs or answering questions, but about articulating desire as that which can never be fully said or fulfilled.[172]

Lacan's theory of desire naturally stems from his theory of language, based on the arbitrary relationship between signifier and signified. The starting point is the radical break that arises between the word and the thing. *Le symbole est le meurtre de la chose.*[173] This 'murder' is committed by symbolic language. It is based on an agreement between speakers, whereby meaning is (only) generated on the basis of the difference between signifiers. This is the distinction between human and animal language. The former is symbolic. It consists of signifiers and is based on convention: 'chair,' 'stoel,' 'chaise,' depending on the culture/language area we find ourselves in. The latter is imaginary and semiotic. It is a form of sign language that conveys a more specific meaning.[174] The index is, in a sense, proto-metonymic. Smoke refers to fire, and a broken branch to a passerby. The icon is proto-metaphorical: the pole refers to a penis, the cave to a vagina. For the human child, the signifier—still according to Lacan—has a structuring function in the parent-child relationship and in the way desire is inscribed in it.

The child has needs, asks for love, and is immersed in a bath of signifiers. It is the mother tongue in which, however, the reference to the third (the Name and the No of the Father, alias the paternal function) must be sufficiently present. After all, the desire of the mother (as the figure of the first great Other) must not be exclusively directed at her child. Only sufficient openness guarantees the possibility of separation with a chance of one's own desire, albeit in permanent dependence on the desire of the Big Other (by extension/in general). Immediately, in this Lacanian logic, the chicken-and-egg question of parentification is 'resolved.' Desire is dialectical and cannot be defined on the basis of simple causality. The subject/child has needs, transforms them into questions, and is driven by desire. The Big Other mirrors this process, makes demands, raises questions, and the subject tries to guess what exactly is expected/desired by the Big Other. This relationship is never symmetrical. Desire remains undefined on both sides and is marked by loss and lack.

The child tries to be the object of the Other's desire and to meet their demand in order to secure their love. In doing so, it confronts the parents' opaque, enigmatic fantasy. It is faced with the question *Che vuoi?* (What do you actually want from me?) and this 'sensitivity' is ingrained from the very beginning.[175] One of the most fundamental tasks of parenting/upbringing is perhaps the regulation of pleasure. This means nothing more and nothing less than teaching the child to live with a fact of life, namely, that it cannot have/be everything.

From these theoretical starting points, we can understand how parentification causes a fundamental symbolic disruption in which the child becomes entangled in a form of Mission Impossible. Desire and subjectivity become entangled in the process. Lacan's mirror stage is a logical key moment for him when the child identifies with its image in the mirror (or in the eyes of the parent). It derives a coherent self-image from this, which is important for its development.[176] On the other hand, however, this identification is also alienating. The child learns to 'be' what the Big Other (in him) sees. In parentification, the child becomes trapped in the Other's needs. The mirror does not reflect a differentiated subject but an imaginary function: I am what I must be for you: the perfect child, the emotional caregiver, the saviour. For Lacan, the paternal function must break through the dyadic entanglement between mother and child. He forbids the child to the mother, but also the mother to the child. By thus limiting maternal desire, the deficit is installed and the child gains access to the broader field of language, difference, and social structures. Emotional parentification often occurs in the absence or failure of this paternal function. The child must be the phallus: that imaginary object that makes the Other 'full.'[177] This identification often leads to feelings of guilt, shame and alienation, because the child has sacrificed its own desires and subjectivity.

Lacanian psychoanalysis is not primarily aimed at 'adjustment' or 'healing'[178] but at restructuring the subjective position towards desire and lack. The main goal is to free the subject from the imaginary trap and untangle the symbolic knots. For the parentified patient, this means he must recognise that he is not responsible for the Other's desire or need. Lacan's '*traversée du fantasme*'[179] is simply his formulation for Freud's working-through/*durcharbeiten*: I am not *it* for the Other. He must assume his own desires and detach himself from the roles or functions assigned to him. This liberation can feel like dying or a form of betrayal. After all, the child had built its entire identity and psychological economy around being 'it'/'there' for the Other. Thanks to the analytical process, the parentified child steps out of the phallus's place and begins to speak with its own voice. Even when that voice was silenced long ago.

Notes

1 From earliest to most recent: Kinet (2024, 2025a, 2025b).
2 Particularly in what is referred to as 'the Western world,' this period of dependency is now much longer than it used to be.
3 Freud (1895).
4 Freud (1895); Bion (1974); Anzieu (1985).
5 The protective blanket of imagination and symbolisation (Grotstein 1981).
6 'Threat of annihilation' (Kohut 1971), 'unthinkable anxiety' (Winnicott 1971), 'nameless dread' (Bion 1970).
7 Kinet and Vermote (2005).
8 'Mirroring' (Kohut 1971), 'emotional availability' (Mahler, Pine, and Bergmann 1975), 'attunement' (Stern 1985), 'sensitivity' (Bowlby 1988).
9 Winnicott (1955–1956).
10 Kernberg (1975).
11 Winnicott (1958).
12 Ainsworth et al. (1978); Main and Goldwyn (1995).
13 Mahler, Pine, and Bergmann (1975).
14 Lacan (1949).
15 Klein (1957).
16 Winnicott (1960b).
17 Kinet (1996).
18 Van Haute (2000, pp. 109–111).
19 Lacan (1959–1960).
20 Arno (1995). My translation of 'The eyes of my mother': 'My mother has something. Something dangerous. Something of a seductress. Something of a pain in the neck.'
21 Verhaeghe (2002).
22 Lacan (1956–1957, pp. 240–241).
23 Lacan (1956–1957, p. 69). Dependence is the ultimate 'fact of life' of the human condition and is very frightening, both for those who ask for help and for the care provider. For Winnicott (1950, p. 252), it underlies the '*fear of* WOMAN.' It is the fear of losing oneself and one's subjectivity, whereby, from a Lacanian perspective (in a *sigh*, as it were), we risk disappearing into (the enjoyment of) the Big Other.
24 Dolto (1988).
25 Kinet (2024).
26 Freud (1914).
27 Kinet (2019).
28 Freud (1921).
29 Winnicott (1960b).
30 Freud (1920).
31 Freud (1910).
32 See case study Sam from Intermezzo III.
33 Kets de Vries (2010); Lamia and Krieger (2015); Lampe (2002).
34 Lamia and Krieger (2015).
35 Bowlby (1980).
36 Freud (1915a, 1915b, 1915c).
37 Kets de Vries (2010).
38 Lacan (1955b/1966).
39 In a sense, this dividing line still exists today between the International Psychoanalytic Association and the (Lacanian) World Association of Psychoanalysis. In earlier publications, I elaborated on the distinction between the empiricism of *I*

see and the rationalism of *Je comprends*, which characterise both schools of thought within contemporary psychoanalysis (Kinet 2019). The former remains very open to ethology, primatology, evolutionary biology, neurobiology, and, more generally, scientific observations, while the latter, with its links to philosophy, anthropology, linguistics, literary studies, and critical theory, leans more towards (purely) humanistic inspirations. However, there is the child as we try to reconstruct it from psychoanalytic work with adults, but there is also the child that we can test and observe in the course of its development. The latter often yields findings that call established concepts into question, if not falsifying them. A well-known criticism by Karl Popper is that a theory that can explain everything explains nothing. It is the famous hyperhermeneutics of psychoanalysis that enables it to explain everything and, according to its critics, makes it immune to any form of criticism.

40 Kinet (2024).

41 Both contemporary relational psychoanalysis and trauma and attachment theory are based on his insights, as expressed by Lewis Aron (1996), Philip Bromberg (2011), and Jessica Benjamin (2018), among others.

42 Ferenczi (1932).

43 Borossa (1999, p. 221).

44 Ferenczi (1932, p. 228).

45 Allen, Bateman, and Fonagy (2008).

46 Ferenczi (1931, p. 502).

47 Searles (1965).

48 'The child, in order to preserve at least a part of his psychic life, identifies with the aggressor, introjects him, so that he himself becomes cruel like the aggressor' (Ferenczi 1932, p. 227).

49 Anna Freud (1936).

50 'The mechanism of identification with the aggressor introduces into the ego one of the aggressor's attributes or an entire pattern of behaviour, so that the person threatened transforms himself from the person threatened into the person who makes the threat… This transformation serves as a protection against anxiety. The child, by assuming the attributes of the feared person, seeks to control the situation by becoming like him' (A. Freud, 1936, pp. 109–110).

51 Fairbairn (1943).

52 Fairbairn (1943, p. 64).

53 Fairbairn (1943, p. 67).

54 Fairbairn (1943, p. 66).

55 Kinet (2023); Franckx and Hebbrecht (2023).

56 Kinet (2023): *savoir*/knowledge as in 'see the id' and *faire ainsi*/proceed as follows in an allusion to the name Ferenczi.

57 More on this later.

58 Ferenczi (1930, pp. 118, 160).

59 Chemla (2009 pp. 43–59).

60 De Vleminck (2023) discusses Ferenczi's influence on Winnicott. The references to Ferenczi's German-language publications are all taken from there. Ferenczi speaks literally about the necessity of analysis by an expert. A training analysis must also simply be a therapeutic analysis (Ferenczi 1927, p. 376) because a completed analysis of the analyst is the only reliable basis for a good analytical technique (Ferenczi 1928, p. 397). He emphasises the analyst's role in treatment to fully understand and control inevitable weaknesses and character traits (Ferenczi 1928, p. 382).

61 Ferenczi (1928, p. 383).

62 Ferenczi (1928, p. 390).
63 Ferenczi (1930, p. 489).
64 Ferenczi (1931, p. 503).
65 Hebbrecht (2023).
66 Balint (1937).
67 Freud (1914). Primary narcissism as a stage *before* object love.
68 Balint (1968).
69 Today, the 'basic fault' is more commonly referred to as attachment trauma. In attachment theory, it is understood as a fundamental disruption of the internal working model with which the young child organises its affective world (Bowlby 1969, 1973). Chronic misattunement, affective unavailability, or intrusive caregivers can impair the process of affect regulation and mentalisation, resulting in a fragile or fragmented self-experience (Ainsworth et al. 1978; Fonagy et al. 2002). From a neurobiological perspective, such relational traumatisation leads to permanent dysregulation of the right hemisphere, which is central to early affect communication and stress regulation (Schore 1994). Where attachment theory emphasises the disruption of the internal working model, Balint describes its clinical re-enactment as a regression to an existential relational gap position, in which the patient is less 'willing' than 'receiving' again (Balint, 1968). Both contemporary infant research and relational psychoanalysis understand this rupture as an implicit, non-verbal trace in the self, formed in the early caregiving relationship and later relived in the transference (Beebe and Lachmann 2002; Stern 1985). Thus, the combination of attachment trauma and the *basic fault* forms a theoretical bridge between developmental psychology, neurobiology, and clinical psychoanalysis: the former describes *how* it is formed, the latter *how* it is clinically relived and processed. See also below.
70 Main and Solomon (1986).
71 van der Kolk (2014).
72 Fernando (2009).
73 Sklar (2012); Balint (1968, p. 138).
74 Freud and Ferenczi (1996, p. xxxv, note 14).
75 Young-Bruehl (2002, p. 412).
76 Goethe (1832, p. 269).
77 If the patient never received a word of appreciation or affirmation as a child, the therapist's sustained supportive and encouraging attitude provides a corrective emotional experience: this new 'object relationship' is internalised and strengthens (self-)confidence. In turn, however, this can lead to dependence: ultimately, the need must be *analysed* rather than satisfied.
78 Rockland (1989).
79 See my aforementioned trilogy on psychodynamic psychiatry.
80 Kinet and Vermote (2005).
81 Kinet (2024).
82 Kinet (1996).
83 Cambien (1988).
84 Which she later reinterprets in her work as envy.
85 Symington (1986, pp. 303–304).
86 Phenomenologically appearing as hatred and envy.
87 Winnicott (1969a pp. 462–463).
88 Winnicott (1956).
89 Winnicott (1960a, p. 54).
90 Winnicott (1969b, pp. 255–257).
91 Winnicott, (1962, p. 61).

92 In the psychoanalytic space, being able/allowed/daring to be 'silent' can have a healing effect on the analysand. There is no need for verbal interpretation. This is the feminine element in psychoanalysis, where *being* is more important than *doing* (see Winnicott 1958, pp. 29–30; Winnicott 1971, pp. 80–81).
93 Winnicott (1945, p. 154).
94 These views are very much in line with the concept *of 'violence fondamentale'* that Jean Bergeret proposes as an alternative to Freud's death drive.
95 Winnicott (1939, p. 88).
96 Winnicott (1963b).
97 Winnicott (1986).
98 I quote Klein (1935 p. 285, my italics):

> The object-world of the child in the first two or three months of life could be described as consisting of hostile and persecuting, or else of gratifying parts and portions of the real world. Before long, the child perceives more and more of the whole person of the mother, and this more realistic perception extends to the world beyond the mother. *The fact that a good relationship with its mother and the external world helps the baby to overcome its early paranoid anxieties sheds light on the importance of its earliest experiences…* only since we know more about the nature and contents of its early anxieties, and *the continuous interplay between its actual experiences and its fantasy life, can we fully understand why the external factor is so important.*

99 Winnicott (1954, p. 281).
100 Winnicott (1954, pp. 285–286).
101 Monjauze (1999).
102 Winnicott (1968a).
103 'Phantasy is (in the first instance) the mental corollary, the psychic representative of instinct. There is no impulse, no instinctual urge or response which is not experienced as unconscious phantasy' (Klein 1959, p. 251). See also Cambien (1988).
104 Klein (1946).
105 Depending on the theory, this refers to a 'self-other-affect triad' (Kernberg 1984), proto-narrative envelopes/schemas of togetherness (Stern 1985), an 'inner working model' (Bowlby 1988), a certain attachment pattern (Main and Goldwyn 1995), a cognitive schema (Bucci 1999), and so on, which (in the form of a basic transference) determine our way of being in the world.
106 Thys (2010). What follows is largely based on his analysis of envy and reparation.
107 Hinshelwood (1991, p 168).
108 Compare with the difference between the imaginary Ideal Self and the symbolic Self-ideal: *being* ideal vs *having* an ideal.
109 Freud (1915a, p. 43).
110 Etchegoyen, Lopez, and Rabih (1987), Rosenfeld (1971).
111 Lacan (1964b).
112 This envious parentification can occur, for example, in the narcissistic personality (as described by Otto Kernberg [1975]) with its defensive bastion of the grandiose self.
113 Klein (1937, p. 308).
114 Klein (1937, p. 336).
115 Winnicott (1960b p. 145).
116 Bion (1962b pp. 89–94; 1963, pp. 90–97).

117 Bion (1962b pp. 6–12).
118 Thys (2015).
119 Bion (1959).
120 Bion (1962b, p. 7); Ogden (1986).
121 Kernberg (1975, p. 243).
122 Kernberg (1984).
123 'The pathological superego typically includes archaic and sadistic introjects that attack the ego' (Kernberg, 2004, p. 60).
124 Kernberg (1975, p. 236).
125 Rosenfeld (1964); Bernardi and Eidlin (2018).
126 Kernberg et al. (2008, p. 98).
127 Kohut (1971).
128 Kohut (1977).
129 Bowlby (1980).
130 Bowlby (1973, p. 264).
131 Mikulincer and Shaver (2016).
132 Main and Goldwyn (1995).
133 Nicolai (2009, 2010).
134 Shaver, Belsky, and Brennan (2000).
135 Fonagy et al. (1991).
136 van IJzendoorn (1994).
137 Hesse (2008).
138 Beebe and Lachman (2002).
139 Beebe and Lachman (2002).
140 Van IJzendoorn and Bakermans-Kranenburg (2008).
141 Schuengel (1997), Solomon and George (1999), Lyons-Ruth and Jacobvitz (1999).
142 Cicchetti and Toth (1995).
143 Lyons-Ruth (1998, 2002).
144 MacDonald et al. (2008).
145 Nicolai (2010).
146 Partly derived from Nicolai (2010).
147 Wallin (2007).
148 Fonagy et al. (2015); Fonagy and Campbell (2019).
149 Fonagy et al. (2002).
150 Van IJzendoorn and Bakermans-Kranenburg (2019).
151 Main, Kaplan, and Cassidy (1985); Van IJzendoorn (1994).
152 Bakermans-Kranenburg, van IJzendoorn, and Juffer (2003); Slade (2005), Berlin, Zeanah, and Lieberman 2016).
153 Mahler, Pine, and Bergmann (1975).
154 Beebe, Lachman, and Markese (2012); Beebe and Lachman (2017).
155 Stern (1985).
156 Tronick et al. (1978).
157 Tronick (2007).
158 Schore (1994, 2001, 2021).
159 Schore (2001).
160 Clark et al. (2021).
161 Kundakovic and Champagne (2014).
162 Schore (2019, p. 22).
163 Mitchell (1988), Mitchell and Aron (1999), Benjamin (1995, 2004).
164 Schore (2019, pp. 35–42).
165 Schore (2019, p. 44).
166 Schore (2019, p. 63).

167 Schore (2019, p. 215).
168 'La demande déborde toujours les satisfactions particulières qui pourraient y répondre. C'est dans cet excès que naît le désir' Lacan (1954–1955, p. 223).
169 Van Haute (2000).
170 Need becomes demand the moment it is articulated in language. From then on, it is no longer a simple need, but is addressed to the Other. This demand is twofold: a demand for an object but also a demand for love. Lacan (1953–1954, p. 235).
171 'An instinct can never be eradicated; only the channels by which it operates can be changed' (Freud (915d, p. 123).
172 'The question can be satisfied with an answer. The demand, even when satisfied in its object, remains insatiable, because it is in essence a demand for love' (Lacan 1964a, p. 235) or 'The demand for love, which goes beyond need, engenders desire, which can never be satisfied by any object' Lacan (1966b, p. 690).
173 Lacan (1953, p. 319).
174 Peirce (1994).
175 For more on this *Che vuoi?* and the primal seduction in Jacques Lacan and Jean Laplanche, see Kinet (2025c).
176 Lacan (1949) introduced the imaginary and the mirror stage in the context of ethological findings by, for example, Nico Tinbergen and Konrad Lorenz, where the sight of a fellow species has a propulsive effect on one's own development. Lionel Bailly (2012) makes a striking comparison with the (in a sense premature) unification of Germany, which lifted the entire country to a higher level.
177 'The phallus, signifier of the desire of the Other, marks the place of lack' (Lacan (1966b, p. 693).
178 Lacan (1955a, p. 325).
179 Lacan (1966–1967).

References

Ainsworth, M. D. S., Blehar, M. C., Waters, E., Wall, S. (1978). *Patterns of Attachment: A Psychological Study of the Strange Situation*. Hillsdale, NJ: Erlbaum.

Allen J. G., Bateman W., and Fonagy P. (2008). *Mentaliseren in de klinische praktijk*. Amsterdam: Uitgeverij Nieuwezijds.

Anzieu, D. (1985). *The Skin Ego* (C. Turner, trans.). New Haven, CT: Yale University Press, 1989.

Aron, L. (1996). *A Meeting of Minds: Mutuality in Psychoanalysis*. Hillsdale, NJ: Analytic Press.

Arno. (1995). Les yeux de ma mère [Song]. On *À la française* [Album]. Delabel.

Bailly, L. (2012). *Lacan: A Beginner's Guide*. New York: Simon and Schuster.

Bakermans-Kranenburg, M. J., van IJzendoorn, M. H., and Juffer, F. (2003). Less is more: Meta-analyses of sensitivity and attachment interventions in early childhood. *Psychological Bulletin*, 129 (2), 195–215. doi:10.1037/0033-2909.129.2.195

Balint, M. (1937). *Primary Love and Psycho-analytic Technique*. London/New York: Routledge, 2013.

Balint, M. (1968). *The Basic Fault: Therapeutic Aspects of Regression*. London: Tavistock.

Beebe, B. and Lachman, F. (2002). *Infant Research and Adult Treatment*. New York: Analytic Press.

Beebe, B. and Lachmann, F. (2017). *The Mother–Infant Interaction Picture Book: Origins of Attachment*. New York: Norton.

Beebe, B., Lachmann, F. M., and Markese, S. (2012). On the origins of disorganized attachment and internal working models: Paper II. An empirical microanalysis of 4-month mother–infant interaction. *Psychoanalytic Dialogues*, 22 (4), 352–374. doi:10.1080/10481885.2012.679606

Benjamin, J. (2018). *Beyond Doer and Done to: Recognition Theory, Intersubjectivity, and the Third*. New York: Routledge.

Bergeret, J. (1974). *La violence fondamentale: Essai de psychopathologie du lien social*. Paris: Dunod.

Berlin, L. J., Zeanah, C. H., and Lieberman, A. F. (2016). Prevention and intervention programs to support early attachment security. In J. Cassidy and P. R. Shaver (eds), *Handbook of Attachment* (3rd edn, pp. 739–758). New York: Guilford.

Bernardi, R., and Eidlin, M. (2018). Thin-skinned or vulnerable narcissism and thick-skinned or grandiose narcissism: Similarities and differences. *The International Journal of Psychoanalysis*, 99 (2), 291–313. doi:10.1080/00207578.2018.1425599

Bion, W. R. (1959). Attacks on linking. *International Journal of Psycho-Analysis*, 40 (5–6),308–315.

Bion, W. R. (1962). *Learning from Experience*. London: Heinemann.

Bion, W. R. (1963). *Elements of Psycho-analysis*. London: Heinemann.

Bion, W. R. (1970). *Attention and Interpretation*. London: Karnac.

Bion, W. R. (1974). *Bion's Brazilian Lectures*. London: Karnac, 1990.

Borossa, J. (1999). Therapeutic relations: Sándor Ferenczi and the British independents. In E. Caldwell (ed.), *Winnicott and the psychoanalytic tradition* (pp. 141–164). London/New York: Routledge, 2018.

Bowlby, J. (1969). *Attachment and Loss: Vol. 1. Attachment* (2nd edn). New York: Basic Books, 1982.

Bowlby, J. (1973). *Attachment and Loss: Vol. 2. Separation: Anxiety and Anger*. New York: Basic Books.

Bowlby, J. (1980). *Attachment and Loss: Vol. 3. Loss: Sadness and Depression*. New York: Basic Books.

Bowlby, J. (1988). *A Secure Base. Clinical Applications of Attachment Theory*. London/New York: Routledge.

Bromberg, P. M. (2011). *The Shadow of the Tsunami and the Growth of the Relational Mind*. New York: Routledge.

Bucci, W. (1999). *Psychoanalysis and Cognitive Science: A Multiple Code Theory*. New York: Guilford Press.

Cambien, J. (1988). Fantasie in het werk van Melanie Klein. *Tijdschrift voor Psychotherapie*, 14, 258–268.

Chemla, P. (2009). Neutralité malveillante. *La Clinique lacanienne*, 15, 43–59.

Cicchetti, D. and Toth, S. (1995). Developmental psychopathology perspective on child abuse and neglect. *Journal of the American Academy of Child and Adolescent Psychiatry*1995; 34 (5), 541–565.

Clark, E. L., Jiao, Y., Sandoval, K., and Biringen, Z. (2021). Neurobiological implications of parent–child emotional availability: A review. *Brain Sciences*, 11 (8), 1016. doi:10.3390/brainsci11081016

De Vleminck, J. (2023). Ferenczi met Winnicott over het infantiele trauma. In: Franckx, C. and Hebbrecht, M. *Het kinderlijk trauma. Verloren tussen tederheid en passie* (pp. 221–237). Antwerpen/'s-Hertogenbosch: Gompel and Svacina.

Dolto, F. (1988). *Quand les parents se séparent* (I. de Angelino, coauthor.). Paris: Seuil.

Etchegoyen, H., Lopez, B. and Rabih, M. (1987), Envy and how to interpret it. *International Journal of Psycho-Analysis*, 68, 49–61.

Fairbairn, W. R. D. (1943). The repression and the return of bad objects. *Psychoanalytic Studies of the Personality* (pp. 59–81). London: Tavistock, 1952.

Ferenczi, S. (1927). Die Anpassung der Familie an das Kind. *Bausteine zur Psychoanalyse, Band III: Arbeiten aus den Jahren 1908–1933* (pp. 347–366). Bern/Stuttgart: Hans Huber, 1964.

Ferenczi, S. (1928). Die Elastizität der psychoanalytischen Technik. *Bausteine zur Psychoanalyse, Band III: Arbeiten aus den Jahren 1908–1933* (pp. 380–398). Bern/ Stuttgart: Hans Huber, 1964.

Ferenczi, S. (1930). Relaxationsprinzip und Neokatharsis. *Bausteine zur Psychoanalyse, Band III: Arbeiten aus den Jahren 1908–1933* (pp. 468–489). Bern/Stuttgart: Hans Huber, 1964.

Ferenczi, S. (1931). Kinderanalysen mit Erwachsenen. *Bausteine zur Psychoanalyse, Band III: Arbeiten aus den Jahren 1908–1933* (pp. 490–510). Bern/Stuttgart: Hans Huber, 1964.

Ferenczi, S. (1932). *The Clinical Diary of Sándor Ferenczi* (M. Balint, ed.; M. Dupont, trans.). Cambridge, MA: Harvard University Press, 1988.

Fernando, J. (2009). *The Processes of Defence: Trauma, Drives, and Reality—A New Synthesis.* London: Karnac.

Fonagy, P., Steele, M., Steele, H., Moran, G. S., and Higgitt, A. C. (1991). The capacity for understanding mental states: The reflective self in parent and child and its significance for security of attachment. *Infant Mental Health Journal*, 12 (3), 201–218. doi:10.1002/1097-0355(199123)12:3

Fonagy, P., Gergely, G., Jurist, E., and Target, M. (2002). *Affect Regulation, Mentalization, and the Development of the Self.* New York: Other Press.

Fonagy, P., Luyten, P., and Allison, E. (2015). Epistemic petrification and the restoration of epistemic trust: a new conceptualization of borderline personality disorder and its treatment. *Journal of Personality Disorders*, 29 (5), 575–609. doi:10.1521/ pedi.2015.29.5.575

Fonagy, P., and Campbell, C. (2019). Mentalizing, attachment and epistemic trust: how psychotherapy can promote resilience. *Journal of Child Psychotherapy*, 45 (1), 91–108. https://discovery.ucl.ac.uk/id/eprint/1574378

Franckx, C. and Hebbrecht, M. (eds) (2023). *Het kinderlijk trauma. Verloren tussen tederheid en passie.* Antwerpen; 's-Hertogenbosch: Gompel and Svacina.

Freud, A. (1936). *The Ego and the Mechanisms of Defence. The Writings of Anna Freud (Vol. II)*. New York: International Universities Press, 1974.

Freud, S. (1895). *Het ontwerp* (G. Van de Vijver and F. Geerardyn, vert. and inl.). Gent, België: Idesça, 1992.

Freud, S. (1910). A special type of choice of object made by men (Contributions to the psychology of love I). In *S. E.* (Vol. 11, pp. 165–175). London: Hogarth.

Freud, S. (1914). On narcissism: An introduction. In *S. E.* (Vol. 14, pp. 73–102). London: Hogarth, 1957.

Freud, S. (1915a). Driften en hun lotgevallen. In *Werken* (Vol. 7, pp. 17–44). Amsterdam: Boom, 2006.

Freud, S. (1915b). Repression. In *S. E.* (Vol. 14, pp. 143–158). London: Hogarth.

Freud, S. (1915c). The unconscious. In *S. E.* (Vol. 14, pp. 159–215). London: Hogarth, 1961.

Freud, S. (1915d). Instincts and their vicissitudes. In *S. E.* (Vol. 14, pp. 109–140). London: Hogarth.

Freud, S. (1920b). Beyond the pleasure principle. In *S. E.* (Vol. 18, pp. 1–64). London: Hogarth, 1961.

Freud, S. (1921). Group psychology and the analysis of the ego. In *S. E.* (Vol. 18, pp. 65–143). London: Hogarth, 1955.

Freud, S., and Ferenczi, S. (1996). *The Correspondence of Sigmund Freud and Sándor Ferenczi* (E. Falzeder, E. Brabant, and P. Giampieri-Deutsch, eds). Cambridge, MA/London: The Belknap Press of Harvard University Press.

Goethe, J.W. (1832). 'Faust – Deel Twee'. In: J.W. von Goethe (1982). *Faust*. Deel Een en Twee. Amsterdam: Wereldbibliotheek.

Grotstein, J. (1981). Who is the dreamer who dreams the dream and who is the dreamer who understands it?*Do I Dare Disturb the Universe?* (pp. 110–145). London: Karnac.

Hebbrecht, M. (2023). Het klinische dagboek van Sándor Ferenczi. Psychoanalyse van trauma. In Franckx, C. and Hebbrecht, M., *Het kinderlijk trauma. Verloren tussen tederheid en passie* (pp. 157–170). Antwerpen/'s Hertogenbosch: Gompel and Svacina.

Hesse, E. (2008). The Adult Attachment Interview: Protocol, method of analysis, and empirical studies. In J. Cassidy and P. R. Shaver (eds), *Handbook of Attachment: Theory, Research, and Clinical Applications* (2nd edn, pp. 552–598). New York: Guilford.

Hinshelwood, R. D. (1991). *A Dictionary of Kleinian Thought*. London: Free Association Books.

Kernberg, O. F. (1975). *Borderline Conditions and Pathological Narcissism*. New York: Jason Aronson.

Kernberg, O. F. (1984). *Severe Personality Disorders: Psychotherapeutic Strategies*. New Haven, CT: Yale University Press.

Kernberg, O. F. (2004). *Aggression in Personality Disorders and Perversions*. New Haven, CT: Yale University Press.

Kernberg, O. F., Yeomans, F. E., Clarkin, J. F., and Levy, K. N. (2008). Transference focused psychotherapy: Overview and update. *International Journal of Psychoanalysis*, 89 (3), 601–620. doi:10.1111/j.1745-8315.2008.00046.x

Kets de Vries, M. (2010). *Leadership Coaching and the Rescuer Syndrome: How to Manage Both Sides of the Couch*. Faculty and Research and Working Paper. Geneve: INSEAD.

Kinet, M. (1996). Weerzien met...Melanie Klein. *Tijdschrift voor Psychotherapie*, 22, 197–211.

Kinet, M. and Vermote, R. (eds) (2005). *Mentalisatie*. Antwerpen/Apeldoorn: Garant.

Kinet, M. (2019). Enkele oedipale variaties. Van Darwin tot Lacan. In Kinet, M., and Heuves, W. (eds), *Driehoeksverhoudingen. Actuele oedipale variaties* (pp. 51–70). Antwerpen/'s-Hertogenbosch: Gompel and Svacina.

Kinet, M. (2023). Tussen ça voir en faire ainsi. In Franckx, C. and Hebbrecht, M., *Het kinderlijk trauma. Verloren tussen tederheid en passie* (pp. 293–305). Antwerpen/'s-Hertogenbosch: Gompel and Svacina.

Kinet, M. (2024). *Psychoanalytic Principles in Psychiatric Practice. A Remedy by Truth*. London/New York: Routledge.

Kinet, M. (2025a). *Psychoanalytic Psychotherapy in Psychiatric Practice. Premises and Clinical Portraits*. London/New York: Routledge.

Kinet, M. (2025b). *Patient Testimonies of Psychodynamic Psychotherapy. Reported and Recorded.* London/New York: Routledge.

Kinet, M. (2025c). Che Vuoi? Epiloog in enkele contrapunten. In Hebbrecht, M. and De Vleminck, J. (eds) *Verleiding en vertaling. Het enigma van de seksualiteit* (pp. 173–189). Antwerpen/'s-Hertogenbosch: Gompel and Svacina.

Klein, M. (1935). A contribution to the psychogenesis of manic-depressive states. *Love, Guilt and Reparation and Other Works 1921–1945* (pp. 262–289). London: Hogarth, 1975.

Klein, M. (1937). Love, guilt and reparation. In *Love, Guilt and Reparation and Other Works 1921–1945* (pp. 306–343). London: Virago, 1988.

Klein, M. (1946). Notes on some schizoid mechanisms. In *Envy and Gratitude and Other Works 1946–1963* (pp. 1–24). London: Hogarth, 1975.

Klein, M. (1957). Envy and gratitude. In *Envy and Gratitude and Other Works 1946–1963* (pp. 176–235). London: Virago, 1988.

Klein, M. (1959). Our adult world and its roots in infancy. In *Envy and gratitude and other works 1946–1963* (pp. 247–263). London: Virago, 1988.

Kohut, H. (1971). *The Analysis of the Self.* New York: International Universities Press.

Kohut, H. (1977). *The Restoration of the Self.* New York: International Universities Press.

Kundakovic, M., and Champagne, F. A. (2014). Early-life experience, epigenetics, and the developing brain. *Neuropsychopharmacology*, 39 (1), 244–256. doi:10.1038/npp.2013.1559

Lacan, J. (1949). Le stade du miroir comme formateur de la fonction du Je. *Écrits* (pp. 93–100). Paris: Seuil, 1966.

Lacan, J. (1953). Fonction et champ de la parole et du langage en psychanalyse. *Écrits* (pp. 237–322). Paris: Seuil, 1966.

Lacan, J. (1953–1954). *Le Séminaire, Livre I: Les écrits techniques de Freud* (J.-A. Miller, ed.). Paris: Seuil, 1975.

Lacan, J. (1954–1955). *Le Séminaire, Livre II: Le moi dans la théorie de Freud et dans la technique de la psychanalyse* (J.-A. Miller, ed.). Paris: Seuil, 1978.

Lacan, J. (1955a). Variantes de la cure-type. *Écrits* (pp. 323–349). Paris: Seuil, 1966.

Lacan, J. (1955b). La chose freudienne ou Sens du retour à Freud en psychanalyse. *Écrits* (pp. 401–436). Paris: Seuil, 1966.

Lacan, J. (1956–1957). *Le Séminaire, Livre IV: La relation d'objet* (J.-A. Miller, ed.). Paris: Seuil, 1994.

Lacan, J. (1959–1960). *Le Séminaire, Livre VII: L'éthique de la psychanalyse* (J.-A. Miller, ed.). Paris: Seuil, 1986.

Lacan, J. (1964a). *Le Séminaire, Livre XI: Les quatre concepts fondamentaux de la psychanalyse* (J.-A. Miller, ed.). Paris: Seuil, 1973.

Lacan, J. (1964b). *The Four Fundamental Concepts of Psycho-analysis* (A. Sheridan, trans.). New York: Norton, 1977.

Lacan, J. (1966a). *Écrits.* Paris: Seuil.

Lacan, J. (1966b). *Écrits: A selection* (A. Sheridan, trans.). London: Tavistock, 1977.

Lacan, J. (1966–1967). *Le Séminaire, Livre XIV: La logique du fantasme* (J.-A. Miller, ed.). Paris: Seuil, 2023.

Lamia, M. C. and Krieger, M. J. (2015). *The White Knight Syndrome. Rescuing Yourself from Your Need to Rescue Others.* Brattleboro: Echo Point Books.

Lampe, P. (2002). *Het Moeder Theresasyndroom, het persoonlijke motief in de hulpverlening*. Amsterdam: Boom.

Lyons-Ruth, K. (1998). Implicit relational knowing: its role in development and psychoanalytic treatment. *Infant Mental Health Journal*, 19, 282–289.

Lyons-Ruth, K., and Jacobvitz, D. (1999). Attachment disorganization: Unresolved loss, relational violence, and lapses in behavioral and attentional strategies. In J. Cassidy and P. R. Shaver (eds), *Handbook of Attachment: Theory, Research, and Clinical Applications* (pp. 520–554). New York: Guilford.

Lyons-Ruth, K. (2002). Dissociation and the parent-infant dialogue: a longitudinal perspective from attachment research. *Journal of the American Psychoanalytical Association*, 51 (3), 884–911.

MacDonald, H. Z., Beeghly, M., Grant-Knight, W., Augustyn, M., Woods, R. W., Cabral, H., and Frank, D. A. (2008). Longitudinal association between infant disorganized attachment and childhood posttraumatic stress symptoms. *Development and Psychopathology*, 20 (2), 493–508. doi:10.1017/S0954579408000243

Mahler, M., Pine, S. and Bergmann, A. (1975). *The Psychological Birth of the Human Infant*. New York: Basic Books.

Main, M., Kaplan, N., and Cassidy, J. (1985). *Security in Infancy, Childhood, and Adulthood: A Move to the Level of Representation. Monographs of the Society for Research in Child Development*, 50 (1–2), 66–104.

Main, M., and Solomon, J. (1986). Discovery of a new, insecure-disorganized/disoriented attachment pattern. In T. B. Brazelton and M. Yogman (eds), *Affective Development in Infancy* (pp. 95–124). Norwood: Ablex.

Main, M. and Goldwyn, S. (1995). Interview-based adult attachment classification: related to infant-mother and infant-father attachment. *Developmental Psychology*, 19, 237–223.

Mikulincer, M., and Shaver, P. R. (2016). *Attachment in Adulthood: Structure, Dynamics, and Change* (2nd edn). New York: Guilford.

Mitchell, S. A. (1988). *Relational Concepts in Psychoanalysis: An Integration*. Cambridge, MA: Harvard University Press.

Mitchell, S. A., and Aron, L. (Eds.). (1999). *Relational Psychoanalysis: The Emergence of a Tradition*. New York: The Analytic Press.

Monjauze, M. (1999). *La part alcoolique du soi: la prise en charge clinique des patients alcooliques*. Paris: Dunod.

Nicolai, N. (2009). Gedesorganiseerde gehechtheid. Van babyonderzoek tot behandeling. *Tijdschrift voor psychoanalyse*, 15, 16–28.

Nicolai, N. (2010) Parentificatie vanuit gehechtheidsperspectief. In M. Kinet (ed.) *Parentificatie. Als het kind te snel ouder wordt* (pp. 87–106). Antwerpen/Apeldoorn: Garant.

Ogden, T. H. (1986). *The Matrix of the Mind: Object Relations and the Psychoanalytic Dialogue*. New York: Jason Aronson.

Peirce, C. S. (1994), *Peirce on Signs: Writings on Semiotics* (J. Hoopes, ed.) Chapel Hill, NC: University of North Carolina Press.

Rockland, L. H. (1989). *Supportive Therapy. A Psychodynamic Approach*. New York: Basic Books.

Rosenfeld, H. (1964). On the psychopathology of narcissism: A clinical approach. *International Journal of Psychoanalysis*, 45, 332–337.

Rosenfeld, H. (1971), A clinical approach to the psychoanalytic theory of the life and death instinct: an investigation into the aggressive aspects of narcissism. *International Journal of Psycho-Analysis*, 52, 169–178.

Schore, A. N. (1994). *Affect Regulation and the Origin of the Self.* New York: Erlbaum.

Schore, A. N. (2001). Effects of a secure attachment relationship on right brain development, affect regulation, and infant mental health. *Infant Mental Health Journal*, 22 (1–2), 7–66. doi:10.1002/1097-0355(200101/04)22:1

Schore, A. N. (2019). *Right Brain Psychotherapy.* New York: Norton.

Schore, A. N. (2021). *The Development of the Unconscious Mind.* New York: Norton.

Schuengel, C. (1997). Disorganized attachment in infancy: A review of the phenomenon and its implications for clinical practice. *Infant Mental Health Journal*, 18 (1), 3–19. doi:10.1002/(SICI)1097-0355(199721)18:1

Searles, H. F. (1965). The patient as psychiatrist to his analyst. In H. F. Searles, *Collected Papers on Schizophrenia and Related Subjects* (pp. 300–321). New York: International Universities Press.

Shaver, P. R., Belsky, J. A. Y., and Brennan, K. A. (2000). The adult attachment interview and self-reports of romantic attachment: Associations across domains and methods. *Personal Relationships*, 7 (1), 25–43.

Sklar, J. (2012). Regression and new beginnings: Michael, Alice and Enid Balint and the circulation of ideas. *International Journal of Psycho-Analysis*, 93 (4), 1017–1034. doi:10.1111/j.1745-8315.2012.00559.x

Slade, A. (2005). Parental reflective functioning: An introduction. *Attachment and Human Development*, 7 (3), 269–281. doi:10.1080/14616730500245906

Solomon, J., and George, C. (1999). The measurement of attachment security in infancy and childhood. In J. Cassidy and P. R. Shaver (eds), *Handbook of Attachment: Theory, Research, and Clinical Applications* (pp. 287–316). New York: Guilford.

Stern, D. N. (1985). *The Interpersonal World of the Infant.* New York: Basic Books.

Symington, N. (1986). *The Analytic Experience: Lectures from the Tavistock.* London: Free Association Books.

Thys, M. (2010). Tussen nijd en spijt. Parentificatie en reparatie. In M. Kinet (ed.), *Parentificatie. Als het kind te snel ouder wordt* (pp. 59–86). Antwerpen/Apeldoorn: Garant.

Thys, M. (2015) Projectieve identificatie tussen doodsdrift en intersubjectiviteit. *Tijdschrift voor Psychoanalyse*, 2, 83–97.

Tronick, E., Als, H., Adamson, L., Wise, S., and Brazelton, T. B. (1978). The infant's response to entrapment between contradictory messages in face-to-face interaction. *Journal of the American Academy of Child Psychiatry*, 17 (1), 1–13.

Tronick, E. (2007). *The Neurobehavioral and Social-Emotional Development of Infants and Children.* New York: Norton.

Van der Kolk, B. A. (2014). *The Body Keeps the Score: Brain, Mind, and Body in the Healing of Trauma.* New York: Viking.

Van Haute, P. (2000). *Tegen de aanpassing.* Nijmegen: SUN.

Van IJzendoorn, M. H. (1994). *Gehechtheid tussen ouders en kinderen.* Houten: Bohn Stafleu Van Loghum.

Van IJzendoorn, M. H. and Bakemans-Kranenburg, M. H. (2008). The distribution of adult attachment representations in clinical groups. Metanalytic search for patterns

in attachment. In H. Steele and M. Steele (eds), *Clinical Applications of the Adult Attachment Interview* (pp. 69–96). New York: Guilford.
Van IJzendoorn, M. H., and Bakermans-Kranenburg, M. J. (2019). Bridging the transmission gap: What attachment measures can teach us. *Attachment and Human Development*, 21 (4), 402–409.
Verhaeghe, P. (2002). *Over normaliteit en andere afwijkingen*. Leuven/Leusden: Acco.
Wallin, D. (2007). *Attachment in Psychotherapy*. New York: Guilford.
Winnicott, D. W. (1939). Aggression and its roots. In C. Winnicott, R. Shepherd, and M. Davis (eds), *Deprivation and Delinquency* (pp. 86–94). London: Tavistock, 1984.
Winnicott, D. W. (1945). Primitive emotional development. *Through Paediatrics to Psycho-analysis* (pp. 145–156). London: Karnac, 1992.
Winnicott, D. W. (1947). Hate in the countertransference. *Through Paediatrics to Psycho-analysis* (pp. 194–203). London: Hogarth, 1958.
Winnicott, D. W. (1950). Some thoughts on the meaning of the word 'democracy.' In C. Winnicott, R. Shepherd, and M. Davis (eds), *Home is Where We Start From: Essays by a Psychoanalyst* (pp. 50–54). London: Penguin, 1986.
Winnicott, D. W. (1951). Transitional objects and transitional phenomena. *International Journal of Psycho-Analysis*, 34, 89–97. *Through Paediatrics to Psycho-analysis* (pp. 229–242). London: Hogarth, 1958.
Winnicott, D. W. (1954). Metapsychological and clinical aspects of regression within the psycho-analytical set-up. *Through Paediatrics to Psycho-analysis* (pp. 278–294). London: Hogarth, 1958.
Winnicott, D. W. (1955–1956). Clinical varieties of transference. *Through Paediatrics to Psycho-analysis* (pp. 295–299). London: Hogarth, 1958.
Winnicott, D. W. (1956). Primary maternal preoccupation. *International Journal of Psycho-Analysis*, 37, 586–595. *Through Paediatrics to Psycho-analysis* (pp. 300–305). London: Hogarth, 1958.
Winnicott, D. W. (1958). The capacity to be alone. *International Journal of Psycho-Analysis*, 39, 416–420. *The Maturational Processes and the Facilitating Environment* (pp. 29–36). London: Hogarth, 1965.
Winnicott, D. W. (1960a). The theory of the parent-infant relationship. *International Journal of Psycho-Analysis*, 41, 585–595. *The Maturational Processes and the Facilitating Environment* (pp. 37–55). London: Hogarth, 1965.
Winnicott, D. W. (1960b). Ego distortion in terms of true and false self. *The Maturational Processes and the Facilitating Environment* (pp. 140–152). London: Hogarth, 1965.
Winnicott, D. W. (1962). Ego integration in child development. In *The Maturational Processes and the Facilitating Environment* (pp. 56–63). London: Hogarth, 1965.
Winnicott, D. W. (1963a). From dependence towards independence in the development of the individual. *The Maturational Processes and the Facilitating Environment* (pp. 83–92). London: Hogarth, 1965.
Winnicott, D. W. (1963b). The development of the capacity for concern. *Bulletin of the Menninger Clinic*, 27 (4), 167.
Winnicott, D. W. (1965). *The Maturational Processes and the Facilitating Environment: Studies in the Theory of Emotional Development*. London: Hogarth.
Winnicott, D. W. (1968a). The use of an object and relating through identifications. *International Journal of Psycho-Analysis*, 49, 585–595.

Winnicott, D. W. (1968b). Communication between infant and mother, and mother and infant, compared and contrasted. *Babies and Their Mothers* (pp. 89–103). Reading, MA: Addison-Wesley, 1987.

Winnicott, D. W. (1969a). Symposium on envy and jealousy. *Psychoanalytic Explorations* (pp. 224–231). London: Karnac, 1989.

Winnicott, D. W. (1969b). The mother–infant experience of mutuality. *Psychoanalytic Explorations* (pp. 215–223). London: Karnac, 1989.

Winnicott, D. W. (1971). *Playing and Reality*. London: Tavistock.

Winnicott, D. W. (1974). Fear of breakdown. *International Review of Psycho-analysis*, 1 (1–2), 103–107.

Winnicott, D. W. (1986). *Holding and Interpretation: Fragment of an Analysis*. London: Karnac, 1989.

Young-Bruehl, E. (2002). A visit to the Budapest School. *The Psychoanalytic Study of the Child*, 57, 411–432.

Chapter 14

Intermezzo VI

Clinical Parentification

In this final intermezzo, I shall present several clinical cases that illustrate the psychodynamics and psychogenesis discussed in the previous chapter. They are drawn from both inpatient and outpatient psychotherapy, ranging from the borderline to the neurotic spectrum, and they are all marked by a factor of manifest or more disguised parentification, depending on whether we are dealing with overt parental needs or with more implicit or subtle expectations and desires.

Kate is in her thirties and has undergone many years of clinical psychotherapy because of a combination of persistent major depression, chronic suicidal ideation, and post-traumatic stress disorder following sexual abuse by an uncle in childhood. Kate was born two months prematurely. She has always known her mother as a very withdrawn and depressive woman who was also hospitalised several times for psychiatric reasons. Her mother frequently absconded, threatening to kill herself. She was taciturn and often scratched her own face until it bled. Kate was constantly alert and sensitively attuned to her mother's moods. She tried to be a good, compliant, and 'easy' child—both to spare and to appease her mother. She also believes she resembles her mother physically and finds it difficult to distinguish between her mother's image and her own reflection in the mirror. Her father is described as highly intellectual, authoritarian, and emotionally distant, attaching excessive importance to academic achievement and social status. The family, as Kate experienced it, was undifferentiated; during a preliminary meeting on the ward, the family therapist felt overwhelmed by them, as if confronted with a many-headed, aggressively charged monster.

Kate was always an extremely quiet, withdrawn child. Time and again, she evoked 'memories' of lying awake in her cot, motionless but conscious, or crying for hours without anyone seeming to hear her. She did well at school, took part in all activities (including youth movements), completed a degree in social care, and worked for several years in that field. Yet she always felt as if she were on autopilot, thinking constantly, 'If only they knew!'—for she was filled with aggressive, murderous, and sadistic fantasies that she kept hidden. In one fantasy, she held her entire family hostage in the cellar with a

DOI: 10.4324/9781003645726-14

flamethrower. Towards the end of therapy, she said, 'Quiet people have a loud mind.'

Kate never really felt she belonged anywhere. She saw herself as 'strange' and 'abnormal.' After years of apparently 'good' functioning, she made a very serious suicide attempt—the proverbial pitcher that goes to the well until it breaks. Since then, her façade has completely collapsed, and her therapy for many years has been dominated by inner devastation. Behind her impassive, mask-like face, a kind of core explosion constantly takes place. She describes these episodes as 'disappearing into fog,' a phenomenological equivalent of what Bion called *attacks on linking*. She often dreams of a post-apocalyptic 'day after,' wandering lost through a devastated, desolate world. From her earliest months, under conditions of basic insecurity and threat, Kate had to develop an *exoskeleton*—an anxious, rigid adaptation to parental and environmental demands. She strove to meet both her mother's and her father's expectations, and that made her an easy prey for an uncle who 'groomed' her during her primary school years. In retrospect, she cannot comprehend how she ever managed to work in the care sector or to become a youth leader. How, she wonders, could she once have been so strong when in adulthood she has required such long-term, total dependence on a clinically psychotherapeutic, 'maternal' environment and mentalising developmental support merely to survive her suicidal drive?

Today, more than ten years later, she remains in outpatient therapy and works as an expert-by-experience, giving talks for patients and teaching in nursing schools. Kate clearly belonged near the borderline spectrum. All the psychodynamic patterns described in the early mother-child relationship were present, and the father's emotional unavailability offered no counterbalance to the black hole (or 'black sun') of Kate's mother.

Sophie was in her late twenties when she was referred by a neurologist for outpatient treatment because of a six-year history of *trichotillomania*. 'I pull hair/her out,' she said (the Dutch word *haar*/hair meaning both 'hair' and 'her'). The symptom began during the final year of secondary school. At that time, she was in a troubled relationship with a man two years her senior. He was extremely demanding and temperamental, and she had to do everything for him—physically and mentally. For several years, she behaved towards his dominance in a slavish and compliant way until, in defiance, she cheated on him: 'I thought, "Fuck you!"' He then hit her and locked her up. She managed to tell her parents and fled from him overnight. He stalked her for more than six months, apparently deeply wounded by her rejection. Her trichotillomania, she said, began as a reaction to the stress of those experiences.

But the pattern of excessive expectations long preceded that. She set a high academic bar, always wanted to be the best, and is now completing a postgraduate master's degree. Her motto is 'Standing still is moving backwards.' She is always in motion, constantly occupied, unable to rest. At the same time, she often feels lonely and cannot bear being alone. 'I have no one,' she says.

At first, she described her parents as kind people who both play golf but do not really suit each other. They do a lot for her. Yet her relationship with her mother is one of 'love-hate.' 'She puts me under enormous pressure. I was my mother's visiting card—she showed me off.' Sophie admires her; her mother is highly ambitious and insists that a woman must be independent, ideally reaching the top of a company. Her mother is having an extramarital affair, of which Sophie is aware but cannot confide in anyone. She sees her as a cold, rational businesswoman who perpetually casts herself as a victim and blames others for every difficulty. Her father, by contrast, she describes as indecisive yet easier to talk to—interested in art, culture, and history—but burdened by alcoholism and marginalised within the family. Her older brother, once a 'problem child,' became a father at eighteen; the family crisis this caused was dramatic, though he has since found his feet.

From early childhood, Sophie suffered from tension headaches like migraines. At primary school, she once cheated on a test and was publicly humiliated, a memory still vivid with shame. She was nervous and wet the bed for years. 'My parents took good care of me, especially materially,' she said. Her mother was often absent; it was mainly her father who spent time with her, though her mother was very strict—she had to finish every meal, even what she disliked. Her mother, slim, attractive, and self-assured, often commented on her daughter's looks and figure, leaving Sophie with deep insecurity and feelings of inferiority.

She attended weekly psychotherapy with me for about two years. I immediately 'read' her trichotillomania as a conversion symptom: the body expressing something unconscious in a linguistic form that requires decoding. In her statement, 'I pull hair out,' I mentally emphasised 'her.' The entire context suggested that, though unaware of it, she harboured long-suppressed anger. Her boyfriend, I felt, was a variant of the narcissistic mother who had treated her as a self-object and controlled her.

As she began to notice within the therapeutic relationship that she was again trying 'to do her best' to meet my expectations, things began to dawn on her. The burden of this effort eventually made her want to 'pull the plug' on therapy. When I linked that phrase to the act of hair-pulling, a light went on. From then on, it became a symbolic key to her problem and provided a recurring interpretive thread for the repetitive patterns in her social and professional life.

As therapy progressed, Sophie began to view her father in a new light. Despite his fine words and love of culture and books, he had been too weak a presence at home, unable to set limits to the imperatives of *mater familias*. She came to feel emotionally abandoned by him and saw him with less idealisation. Later, when she met a 'normal, decent guy' and, despite her mother's disapproval, moved in with him in another province, she concluded her therapy with me. Sometime afterwards, she sent me two cards of thanks—one when she started her own practice, and another announcing the birth of her first child. Her parentification had been primarily of the Kohutian and narcissistic type, though the weakness of the paternal function had also left her exposed as self-object to the pleasure and demands of her mother.

Sandra was a spirited yet delicate woman of forty who sought therapy for anxiety and depression. Shortly before her birth, her paternal grandmother had hanged herself. Sandra always sensed her father's burden of guilt; it was as if the despairing spirit of his mother haunted his mind. He was often absent, withdrawn into his studio, where she would find him quietly weeping. Her mother became hard of hearing at a young age and later became completely deaf. Her older brother was a mischievous rebel who defied all authority. Sandra herself was diligent and perfectionistic, trying to be both an angel and a ray of sunshine in the house. She later admitted how meaningful it was that her father had been prescribed antidepressants from the time of her marriage until his death. She had, in a sense, always been a nurse—and eventually became one professionally. A few years ago, overwhelmed by caring duties, she 'crashed below zero.' She describes herself as highly sensitive.

One childhood memory stands out. She often lay awake at night, unable to sleep because she heard strange noises coming from the neighbours' cellar. It worried her greatly. She repeatedly told her family, nearly screaming 'murder and fire,' but no one ever heard or noticed anything. Only many years later, after new tenants had moved in next door, was the annoying clicking of the central-heating system finally identified as the source.

From our very first conversation, I attributed great significance to this memory. The child's acute listening to noises from the neighbour's cellar symbolised her hyper-attunement to the parents' unconscious needs—her preoccupation with the 'sounds' in their cellar. Her perception of the outer world mirrored her inner one. This sensitivity had led to the construction of a False Self that was bound eventually to collapse. Sandra underwent a long period of clinical psychotherapy. For months, she was utterly disoriented, anxious, clinging, and in constant need of intensive care. Yet alongside her suffering in verbal therapy, she found relief in creative expression in our art studio, located at the heart of the ward and run by a non-therapist artist whose inspiring presence exerts a truly musical influence on everyone.

Now, in outpatient therapy and back at work, Sandra has discovered a passion for clay modelling. Her dream is to craft beautiful, warm (rather than cold and industrial) urns for cremated people and pets—forms that fit their contents as naturally as possible. Death, she says, calls for a fitting container. She has, in a sublimated way, turned her 'high sensitivity' into a gift.

Certain forms of parentification verge on secondary traumatisation. Ordinarily, parents function like oysters, coating the grain of reality with mother-of-pearl. This shell makes a difference—it is Bion's *contact-barrier*, a kind of mental skin. Drives and trauma are mediated by this parental contribution; their symbolising developmental aid tempers affective surges and helps regulate emotional waves. Conversely, when parents fail in this function, the child must mobilise its own mental apparatus to metabolise the parents' drives and traumas. The child responds to the parents' unconscious and unspoken needs, trying to ward them off or repair them. It develops, if necessary, extra antennae—a sixth sense—to anticipate danger and maintain fragile equilibrium. Such children act *proactively* rather than *reactively* towards the presumed needs of an unsafe other. In Sandra's case, this took the form of the wise baby, the False Self, and a reversal of the container-contained relationship. Deep regression was required for her to recover contact with her own idiosyncrasy.

Nicole, in her late twenties, was referred for clinical psychotherapy after a brief psychiatric admission. She initially complained of obsessive thoughts and panic attacks. 'I have a long and beautiful past—very eventful,' she said. The younger of two siblings, she described her father, a technician, as a good dad: strict about order and cleanliness, somewhat authoritarian but calm, humorous, and fun to be with. Her mother, a social worker, she described as emotional, egocentric, theatrical, chaotic, and impulsive—but 'still sweet.'

When Nicole was ten, her father sexually assaulted her friend, the girl next door. Nicole had been secretly infatuated with her brother at the time. Her mother lost all sense of direction, and Nicole felt she had suddenly lost a stable home. What had been an open, lively household, welcoming to the whole neighbourhood, turned into a closed fortress. She was forbidden to ask questions, withdrew to her room, and immersed herself in a fantasy world of books and films—from *Harry Potter* to *The Hunger Games.*

Secondary school was a rollercoaster. Her parents fought frequently and divorced when she was eighteen, forcing her to repeat her final year at art school. She and her older brother moved in with their mother, but there were constant conflicts. The mother's new partner had severe alcohol and drug problems and eventually died of an overdose. After that, her mother drifted from one relationship to another, indulging in promiscuity and visits to swingers' clubs.

Nicole's first breakdown occurred at twenty, leading to six months of day treatment. Afterwards, she pursued higher studies in hospitality management and blossomed socially. She enjoyed nightlife and friendships but was again traumatised when a man she trusted got her drunk and raped her. She shut down once more, withdrawing from everyone and everything, and spent several periods abroad working as an au pair, relishing the sense of being 'a child at home' again.

Nicole was hospitalised for a long time in clinical psychotherapy. She was highly avoidant, seeking contact mainly with patients and staff from other wards. She often wandered through the building or the grounds, with the air of a nomad or gypsy. It took her a long time to build a bond, and she disclosed her story only gradually. When we began to prepare her for day treatment and eventual outpatient psychotherapy, she initially experienced intense feelings of abandonment. Nevertheless, she has since found more stability: she now works part-time, continues her studies, and attends weekly face-to-face sessions.

Here is a recent sequence, verbatim:

> I went to the hairdresser's this week. My mum expects me to dye my hair black with a fringe. She said my haircut was ugly and that I have such a high forehead. I always have to fit a certain image. I don't like being seen as I really am. She has this picture in her head and wants to force me into it. For example, I had to be rebellious, listen to rock music, and dress like a rock chick. I was long under her spell… I always have to go to her, but she never comes to me. She expects too much. She organises parties and I have to take care of everything. When I visit her, I don't even get a cup of coffee, whereas when I come back from my dad's, I return with a suitcase full of food and little gifts he's prepared for me. When I come home from my mum's, I feel exhausted and drained!

Nicole lives alone and struggles with loneliness. Through dating apps, she looks for 'a good man'—tall, strong, and without issues—someone she can lean on. She experiments but keeps her boundaries intact. Yet she has long been fixated on her physiotherapist, who, at one point, began flirting with her. She recently saw him again at a private party where he was behind the bar. She ordered a drink that wasn't available, and he said with a wink, 'I'll fix something for you.' Those words sounded like music to her ears, and she couldn't stop replaying that tune in her mind, even though she knew he was not a good match.

Beyond the Oedipal component, Nicole had long been engulfed by both the oral and narcissistic needs of her mother. Her capacity for mentalisation has now grown to the point where she knows exactly what cards she holds. She recounts almost all her dreams and can now interpret most of them herself. Life, as Kierkegaard said, must be understood backwards, but lived forwards—and Nicole is making progress on both fronts.

Mandy is a young woman in her mid-twenties. She is married and has had three children in quick succession. After the birth of her eldest daughter, she began to be haunted by intrusive images of her children being ill or dead. Following her mother's heart attack, she had similar images of her. She performs various rituals to ward off these obsessive thoughts, but to no avail. That is what brought her to outpatient consultation.

About her mother, she says: 'Mum and I, we're four hands on one belly. I love her to death!'—an unconscious slip, since the saying should be 'two hands on one belly.' She and her mother are *too* close. Her parents divorced when she was thirteen. Her father, a womaniser, used Mandy as an alibi during his amorous escapades. She has affection for him and says they can talk easily; he helps her, especially with practical matters, perhaps out of guilt for his earlier failures as a father.

Her mother, by contrast, has always leaned heavily on Mandy for emotional and romantic support. The parents have been on and off for years, with various other partners coming and going in between. 'Mum tells me everything,' Mandy exclaimed in our first session, her voice cracking on the word 'everything.' At the end of that session, she asked whether her mother could also come to see me. I replied with a question of my own: 'Don't you already share enough?'

In the next session, Mandy confessed she had felt terribly guilty for talking about her mother. Yet she produced abundant material showing how overburdened she felt by her. When her mother calls, she lets the stream of words go in one ear and out the other. 'I feel sorry for her,' she said, 'but I'm really fed up.' She gave many examples of her mother's excessive concern for her grandchildren and the strain this put on Mandy's marriage.

At the end of that session, while paying her fee, she mentioned a dream: she was in prison for a crime she couldn't remember—'as if I'd committed a murder.' We discussed her need to be 'super-sweet' towards her mother. Her mother's words echo in her mind: 'I wouldn't survive without you, darling!' Here, parentification is subtle but unmistakable; Mandy struggles to separate sufficiently from her mother's emotional demands.

Finally, Charles (whom we met in the *Overture*) can speak for himself through excerpts from his weekly psychotherapy sessions:

> I want to grow a beard. The barber trimmed it too short. I was angry, but I said nothing again. Now I feel overwhelmed. I'm furious with the whole world. The anger lingers. I wanted to smash things. I drove around, but it didn't help. I watched a series but couldn't sit still. I took a tranquilliser. I was going mad. I'm tired. I'm always trying to do my best. Also with my wife. I'm indebted to her; financially too. When I've been drinking, I can be nasty. She's sick of my moods. I've got one foot out the door… I'm tired of always struggling. So is she. I'm literally in the red. I'm going bankrupt.
>
> My mother drives me crazy. She can't handle our little daughter. She starts shouting. She can't set boundaries. It's pathetic. She seems afraid of my daughter. She's weak. She talks and talks. She never stops. She gets on my nerves. I keep saying, 'Calm down, calm down!' Everything stresses her out. I feel constantly summoned; help me keep myself upright! I can't respond anymore. I distract myself with my smartphone. I can't look at her. I turn away. I feel on the verge of exploding and collapsing at the same time. I'm also always scanning and reading my wife. I need to leave her in peace more. I smother her.
>
> I like working on my terrarium. Everything else I avoid. I'm so bitter, so angry, so resentful. My worth depends entirely on what I do for others. I try to look after my daughter, work in the garden, and clean the gutters. My life is built around chores. My terrarium, though, that's playtime. As a child, I loved playing outside with other kids—those are my best

memories. Being able, being allowed to be a child. My older brother wasn't there then. When he was around, I had to behave.

I need to stop my private practice. It's too much. I feel like an impostor. I often feel more like a patient than my patients! I'm angry with my parents, my brother, and the whole social sector. It's unfair. I feel deprived, wronged. My wife sometimes doesn't respond. Then I feel lost and insecure. I think I should be hospitalised... My wife's had enough of me. She says I'm childish, irresponsible. I, on the other hand, feel I must work, work, and work again. I don't exist. I get no love, no recognition. I need an emotional address. I have a primal lack. I'm tired of caring for everyone. I haven't sorted out my own mess. I do my best in everything, hoping to earn love. I flog myself. I punish myself. I do forced labour. I wear myself out. I crack the whip over myself...

Every morning, my mother wakes me by pounding on the window when she comes to look after my daughter. Then she comes to my bed to chat. She drives me up the wall. I'm mad with rage and stress. I'm always the one who pays the bill; the unpaid bills of others. My muscles ache all over. I feel it everywhere. I don't want to pay anymore. It's always Charles. The problem's always supposed to be me!

I am very tense, hyperalert. There is a danger... I heard a noise on my daughter's baby monitor. I thought something was wrong. I was anxious and panicky. I threw up earlier because of the tension. No real problems, though. Yet I am in alarm mode. As if my amygdala is on fire. Post-traumatic, surely? ... I only find peace in the evening. All day long, I have to perform, achieve something. It's a mindset. I was already afraid and insecure as a child... I am also having a lot of trouble with dreams again. I dreamed that I was on a weekend away with friends. A comrade was angry with me. I couldn't do anything right. I woke up tired. I had a sweating attack. It's always the same theme. I'm not doing well. It's not working... There was a tiger in my basement. I had accidentally let it loose.... My mother panics about everything. She gets on my nerves. It annoys me to death. I reflect, and she doesn't. We all have problems, but she never seems to wonder if this has anything to do with her.

I urged my wife to see the GP. She has her problems, too. She's also a patient... I can't get above zero. I had a dream. I was in a sheltered workshop with two guys with disabilities. I pretended to be a supervisor but was secretly one of the patients. Then I was in a prison cell, on a wooden bed with only a threadbare blanket. It looked like a construction site. Then I was walking through a city street known for drugs. Someone spoke to me. The streets turned to rivers. I was drowning and lost at the same time. Then I was at my father's funeral; I've dreamed that often. The whole family was there. We had to eat cake, but I'm glucose-intolerant. A woman came in with an illegitimate child. Perhaps I'd like to be that child. On my father's side, the family is rich, or pretends to be. They

> rummage through each other's stuff. They're vultures, picking at my father's artworks. He left me nothing. I had to learn to shave on my own. I was angry. I shouted. My father struts around like a big shot, telling stories about important people; as if his children weren't the most important of all!

One last fragment:

> I dreamt that my father and my eldest brother were in prison. I was interrogated, and I revealed everything they had done wrong. Symbolically, it is quite clear. My father wasn't there. He acted important and interesting everywhere, and I had to do all the work at home… My wife is doing better, but I miss sexual contact. I think sex is important. My wife won't let me drink any beer anymore. I feel a lot of bitterness and anger.

In a famous scene from *The Shining* starring Jack Nicholson, Nicholson's character keeps repeating the same sentence: 'All work and no play makes Jack a dull boy.' Charles associates with a kind of primal rage that he carries around with him. He is full of explosives but is afraid of blowing up relationships. He uses this explosive energy as fuel to work. Sometimes he cannot stop, for example, tidying up or working on his terrarium. When he works for someone else, he is furious, and when he wants to relax, he feels guilty. For him to work hard is the better option, because at least then he is productive…

Chapter 15

Final

Fatefully Yours!

As in my book on psychodynamic psychiatry, I will conclude this epilogue on a mixed philosophical and psychoanalytical note.[1] The pre-Socratic philosopher Heraclitus is credited with the following famous statement: character is fate.[2] This ancient Greek wisdom holds that our destiny is not outside us but *within* us. In psychoanalysis, this intuition is revived in Freud's idea that we are not determined by gods or other supernatural forces, but by our unconscious drives and desires. In his view, our character is a kind of compromise formation: the visible structure that, as it were, seals the conflicts between the id, ego, superego, and reality. For example, in the case of the compulsive personality, the characteristic thriftiness, orderliness, and stubbornness are simply a petrification of earlier libidinal fixations.[3] Character is actually our solidified history that exerts its 'fatal' effect on us.

Freud's research into repetition and repetition compulsion[4] also clarifies why our character offers us coherence, structure, and stability on the one hand, but on the other hand becomes a prison from which we would like to free ourselves. Our character is the way in which the unconscious has organised its pattern of repetition into a form of identity. It protects, but at the same time restricts: it prevents chaos, but keeps us locked in our characteristic stereotypes. If we ascend to the post-Socratic Aristotle, we are what we repeatedly do.[5] Viewed in this way, character is not an innate but an acquired destiny. It is a blueprint of past 'solutions' to sometimes existential pain.

Nietzsche saw our character as a form of necessity: become who you are.[6] For him, freedom did not lie in escaping this necessity, but in consciously and stylishly affirming one's own form by embracing one's own fate: *amor fati*.[7] Psychoanalysis shares this tragic perspective: healing does not mean erasing repetition, but learning to think and often even affirming what you do over and over again. In that respect, Freud was a modern tragedian: man is doomed to repeat his past… until he understands it.

Jacques Lacan later formulated this as follows: '*Le destin du sujet, c'est son fantasme.*' The fate of the subject is his fantasy. In his terminology, the fantasy structures the relationship between the subject and his desire. It is an

DOI: 10.4324/9781003645726-15

unconscious and fundamental construction that determines the way of loving, of suffering, of desiring or, more generally, of understanding the world. This fantasy serves to conceal the lack, because without it the subject would be overwhelmed by fear.[8] He later clarifies this general statement even further. The fantasy becomes the pillar around which the patient's fate revolves and which determines his particular trajectory.[9]

Wilfred Bion perhaps offers a slightly more hopeful twist. For him, fate is that which cannot be thought.[10] Only when affects are not contained do they petrify into character. Psychotherapy attempts to 'liquidate' this solidification: emotions that were once too threatening can then start to move again. Winnicott also described something similar with his idea of the True and False Self.[11] The character of the (so-called) 'well-adjusted' patient is often a survival construct. It is a False Self that shields the true desire. For him, breaking through character patterns therefore does not mean the destruction of identity, but above all the restoration of (play) space.

Take a patient who is constantly at the service of others, saying, 'That's just the way I am, I can't help it.' In analysis, it turns out that this 'not being able to help it' was the survival strategy of a child who only received love by caring for others. His character (helpful, responsible, tireless) is his fate: a repetition of his earlier care for his needy parent. When he learns to recognise this pattern, his character is not abolished, but becomes more differentiated: caring can now be chosen more freely. Fate becomes history, compulsion becomes style. Recognition and acknowledgement open the door to change. When people learn to read their character as the text of their past, they can also rewrite this text. Become who you are precisely by (à la Freud) repeating, remembering, and working through.[12] Ultimately, you can even respond to Slavoj Žižek's call: Enjoy your symptom![13]

In psychoanalysis, character is not just description, but also ethics. The question is whether someone lives according to their unconscious truth or goes against it. The 'true character' would be that in which the subject does not deny but bears their own division. In this, psychoanalysis aligns with Socrates' *daimonion*. Rico Sneller refers to this as an inner principle that warns you when you stray too far from yourself.[14] Freedom here is not the opposite of fate, but the awareness of necessity. The subject becomes free when it recognises its repetitions as meaningful rather than blind and compulsive.

After this brief philosophical digression, I will end with both feet firmly planted on clinical ground: parentification as a transgenerational phenomenon. To that end, I will begin (as in my *Overture*) with two one-liners. One: face your demons, or they will raise your children. After all, psychotherapeutic help for the parent also makes a big difference for their child(ren). Two: most people go into therapy because of people who don't go into therapy. The 'identified patient' is usually not the one who is most 'sick' but the one who suffers the most.[15] As Melanie Klein described, the distinction between the paranoid-schizoid and depressive positions implies that in the former, 'evil' is projected outward, whereas in the latter, it is recognised as partly internal, and it is more likely that some kind of psychological help is sought.[16]

Exactly fifty years ago, Selma Fraiberg and her colleagues introduced the concept of 'ghosts in the nursery.'[17] With this metaphor, they referred to unprocessed, traumatic experiences from the parents' childhood that are repeated in the relationship with their own child(ren). These ghosts are uninvited guests at the christening party:[18] the unconscious repetitions of past pain, neglect, or rejection that permeate the young family's emotional climate. Where love and care should prevail, these shadows of the past creep in unnoticed. The mother, who once cried inconsolably herself, cannot bear her child's crying; the father, who was humiliated as a child, feels powerless in the face of his son's dependence. Earlier, reference was also made to ghosts hiding in a kind of crypt.[19] Psychoanalytic insights into transference, repetition, and symbolisation appear applicable to understanding early childhood development and to early-stage intervention. John Bowlby also described how Internal Working Models that are established in the first years of life form the basis for parental sensitivity later on.[20] Mary Main and Erik Hesse even demonstrated that unresolved traumatic experiences in parents (e.g. loss or abuse) are strongly associated with disorganised attachment in their babies.[21] The parent becomes a source of fear instead of a safe haven. This empirically confirms Selma Fraiberg's psychoanalytic intuition: the parent's past becomes the child's present.

More or less simultaneously, Peter Fonagy and Mary Target added an important dimension to the field with their theory of mentalisation.[22] According to them, the intergenerational transmission of trauma is determined not only by affective regulation but also by the parents' reflective ability to understand their own and others' mental states. When a parent can reflect on their own emotions and those of their child, space is created for symbolisation: the 'ghosts' lose their power. Moreover, secure attachment in children correlates strongly with their parents' reflective functioning, regardless of their actual childhood history.[23] In other words, the parent(s)' ability to *think* about the past is more important for the child than their past itself. All these insights together formed the basis for a clinical model that has since become known as 'parent–infant psychotherapy' (PIP).[24] In this form of therapy, the parent-child relationship itself is considered the 'patient.' Together with the parent, the therapist tries to recognise how past fears, losses, or rejections are repeated in the here and now of the interaction with the baby. A kind of positive counterpart to Fraiberg's metaphor also developed: the 'angels in the nursery.' Alicia Lieberman describes how good, caring memories of the parent can also be passed on and have a healing effect on the relationship with the child.[25] These 'angels' represent moments of tenderness, protection, and love that the parent has known (or experienced later in life) and which remain available as a kind of emotional resource. The therapeutic work focuses not only on dispelling the ghosts but also on remembering and anchoring these angels.

The ghosts in the nursery have indeed come a long way clinically: from psychoanalytic observation to John Bowlby's and Peter Fonagy's empirically based developmental psychology and from symbol to Allan Schore's neuropsychoanalytically studied mechanism. Through epigenetic transmission, trauma and parentification even leave chromosomal traces that can be activated in less favourable circumstances.[26] Nevertheless, the therapeutic task remains unchanged: understanding and working through the parent's inner history. This is crucial for the child's well-being. It is common knowledge that ghosts only disappear when they see the light of day, and certainly when they are invited to speak. Only then can the nursery become a place of love and growth. The beneficial effects of psychotherapy extend far beyond the individual psyche. Psychotherapy for the parent can lead to changes in emotion regulation, attachment style, and reflective capacity that ripple out into subsequent generations. Psychotherapy is therefore not only individual but essentially transgenerational: a micro-politics of domestic peace, discovery, and recovery. I am reminded of a Preface from The Future of Humanity philosopher Toby Ord:

> In the months after my daughter was born, the magnitude of everything my parents did for me was fully revealed. I was shocked. I told them; thanked them; apologised for the impossibility of ever repaying them. And they smiled, telling me that this wasn't how it worked; that one doesn't repay one's parents. One passes it on.[27]

Notes

1 Kinet (2024).
2 *Êthos anthrôpōi daimon*. The phrase appears in *Fragments: A Text and Translation* (Heraclitus 1987).
3 Freud (1908).
4 Freud (1914) and Freud (1920) respectively.
5 As he is often quoted in Durant (1926, p. 87).
6 Nietzsche (1908, p. 158).
7 de Vries and Eskens (2017).
8 '*Le fantasme, c'est ce par quoi le sujet se soutient au niveau de son désir*' (Lacan, 1964/1973, p. 185). My transl.: 'Fantasy is what sustains the subject in terms of their desire.'
9 Lacan (1966–1967).
10 Bion (1962).
11 Winnicott (1965).
12 Freud (1914).
13 Žižek (1992). In short: stop trying to become 'normal' or to 'purify' your desire. Instead, recognise and embrace the specific way in which your unconscious speaks. Your *symptom* (as the intersection of *jouissance* with its combination of pleasure and torment) is also your singular truth.

14 Sneller (2020).
15 Ferenchick and Rosenthal (2019).
16 Klein (1935, 1946).
17 Fraiberg, Adelson, and Shapiro (1975).
18 Fraiberg, Adelson, and Shapiro (1975, p. 387).
19 Abraham and Torok (1972).
20 Bowlby (1988).
21 Main and Hesse (1990).
22 Fonagy and Target (2003).
23 Fonagy et al. (1991).
24 Lieberman et al. (2015).
25 Lieberman et al. (2005).
26 Luyten and Fonagy (2015).
27 Ord (2020, p xv).

References

Abraham, N., and Torok, M. (1972). Deuil ou mélancolie: Introjection et incorporation, l'introject et le fantôme. *L'écorce et le noyau* (pp. 125–164). Paris: Flammarion.

Bion, W. R. (1962). *Learning from Experience*. London: Heinemann.

Bowlby, J. (1988). *A Secure Base. Clinical Applications of Attachment Theory*. London/New York: Routledge.

De Vries, A., and Eskens, E. (2017). *Amor fati: Filosoferen tegen het einde – brieven van en voor een stervende filosoof*. Zaltbommel, NL: Vrije Uitgevers.

Durant, W. (1926). *The Story of Philosophy: The Lives and Opinions of the World's Greatest Philosophers*. New York: Simon and Schuster, 2012.

Ferenchick, E., and Rosenthal, D. (2019). Identified patient in family systems theory. In J. Lebow, A. Chambers, and D. C. Breunlin (eds), *Encyclopedia of Couple and Family Therapy* (pp. 1431–1433). Cham: Springer.

Fonagy, P., Steele, M., Steele, H., Moran, G. S., and Higgitt, A. C. (1991). The capacity for understanding mental states: The reflective self in parent and child and its significance for security of attachment. *Infant Mental Health Journal*, 12 (3), 201–218. doi:10.1002/1097-0355(199123)12:3<201:AID-IMHJ2280120307>3.0.CO;2–7

Fonagy, P., and Target, M. (2003). *Psychoanalytic Theories: Perspectives from Developmental Psychopathology*. London: Whurr.

Fonagy, P., Luyten, P., and Allison, E. (2015). Epistemic petrification and the restoration of epistemic trust: a new conceptualization of borderline personality disorder and its treatment. *Journal of Personality Disorders*, 29 (5), 575–609. doi:10.1521/pedi.2015.29.5.575

Fraiberg, S., Adelson, E., and Shapiro, V. (1975). Ghosts in the nursery: A psychoanalytic approach to the problems of impaired mother–infant relationships. *Journal of the American Academy of Child Psychiatry*, 14 (3), 387–421. doi:10.1016/S0002-7138(09)61442–61444

Freud, S. (1908). Character and anal erotism. In *S. E.* (Vol. 9, pp. 167–175). London: Hogarth.

Freud, S. (1914). Remembering, repeating and working-through. In *S. E.* (Vol. 12, pp. 145–156). London: Hogarth, 1958.

Freud, S. (1920). Beyond the pleasure principle. In *S. E.* (Vol. 18, pp. 1–64). London: Hogarth, 1961.

Heraclitus. (1987). *Fragments: A Text and Translation* (T. M. Robinson, ed. and trans.). Toronto: University of Toronto Press.

Kinet, M. (2024) *Psychoanalytic Principles in Psychiatric Practice. A Remedy by Truth*. London/New York: Routledge.

Klein, M. (1935). A contribution to the psychogenesis of manic-depressive states. *The Writings of Melanie Klein: Vol. 1. Love, Guilt and Reparation and Other Works 1921–1945* (pp. 262–289). London: Hogarth, 1975.

Klein, M. (1946). Notes on some schizoid mechanisms. *Envy and Gratitude and Other Works 1946–1963* (pp. 1–24). London: Hogarth, 1975.

Lacan, J. (1964). *Le Séminaire, Livre XI: Les quatre concepts fondamentaux de la psychanalyse* (J.-A. Miller, ed.). Paris: Seuil.

Lieberman, A. F., Padrón, E., Van Horn, P., and Harris, W. W. (2005). Angels in the nursery: The intergenerational transmission of benevolent parental influences. *Infant Mental Health Journal*, 26 (6), 504–520. doi:10.1002/imhj.20071

Lieberman, A. F., Ghosh Ippen, C., and Van Horn, P. (2015). Infant–parent psychotherapy: An evidence-based treatment for early trauma. In J. D. Osofsky (ed.), *Handbook of Infant Mental Health* (3rd edn, pp. 439–449). New York: Guilford.

Luyten, P., and Fonagy, P. (2015). The neurobiology of mentalizing. *Personality Disorders: Theory, Research, and Treatment*, 6 (4), 366–379. doi:10.1037/per0000117

Main, M., and Hesse, E. (1990). Parents' unresolved traumatic experiences are related to infant disorganized attachment status: Is frightened and/or frightening parental behavior the linking mechanism? In M. T. Greenberg, D. Cicchetti, and E. M. Cummings (eds), *Attachment in the Preschool Years* (pp. 161–182). Chicago, IL: University of Chicago Press.

Nietzsche, F. (1908). *Ecce Homo – hoe iemand wordt wat hij is* (P. Hawinkels and P. Beers, vert.). Amsterdam/Antwerpen: de Arbeiderspers, 2005.

Ord, T. (2020). *The Precipice: Existential Risk and the Future of Humanity*. New York: Bloomsbury.

Sneller, R. (2020). Kierkegaard on Socrates' daimonion. *International Journal of Philosophy and Theology*, 81 (1), 87–100. doi:10.1080/21692327.2019.1649602

Winnicott, D. W. (1965). *The Maturational Processes and the Facilitating Environment: Studies in the Theory of Emotional Development*. London: Hogarth.

Žižek, S. (1992). *Enjoy Your Symptom! Jacques Lacan in Hollywood and Out*. London/New York: Routledge.

Bibliography

Abraham, N., and Torok, M. (1972). Deuil ou mélancolie: Introjection et incorporation, l'introject et le fantôme. *L'écorce et le noyau* (pp. 125–164). Paris: Flammarion.
Ackerman, N. W. (1958). *The Psychodynamics of Family Life: Diagnosis and Treatment of Family Relationships.* New York: Basic Books.
Ainsworth, M. D. S., Blehar, M. C., Waters, E., and Wall, S. (1978). *Patterns of Attachment: A Psychological Study of the Strange Situation.* Hillsdale, NJ: Erlbaum.
Aldridge, J. S. and Becker, S. (1993). *Children Who Care: Inside the World of Young Carers.* Loughborough: Loughborough University.
Alexander, P. C. (2014). *Intergenerational Cycles of Trauma and Violence: An Attachment and Family Systems Perspective*, New York: Norton.
Allen J. G., Bateman W., and Fonagy P. (2008). *Mentaliseren in de klinische praktijk.* Amsterdam: Uitgeverij Nieuwezijds.
American Psychiatric Association. (2001). Practice guidelines for the treatment of patients with borderline personality disorder. *Am. J. Psychiatry*, 158, 1–52.
Andolfi, M. (2016). *Multigenerational Family Therapy: Tools, Techniques, and Clinical Strategies.* London/New York: Routledge.
Andolfi, M., Angelo, C., and Nichols, M. P. (1989). *Genograms in Family Assessment.* New York: Norton.
Anzieu, D. (1985). *The Skin Ego* (C. Turner, trans.). New Haven, CT: Yale University Press, 1989.
Arno. (1995). Les yeux de ma mère [Song]. On *À la française* [Album]. Delabel.
Aron, L. (1996). *A Meeting of Minds: Mutuality in Psychoanalysis.* Hillsdale, NJ: Analytic Press.
Aronovsky, D. (Director) (2000). *Requiem for a Dream.* Universal Pictures.
Asen, E., and Fonagy, P. (2017). *Mentalization-Based Treatment for Families.* New York: Guilford.
Baggett, E., Shaffer, A., and Muetzelfeld, H. (2015). Father-daughter parentification and young adult romantic relationships among college women. *Journal of Family Issues*, 36 (6), 760–783. doi:10.1177/0192513X13499759
Bailly, L. (2012). *Lacan: A Beginner's Guide.* New York: Simon and Schuster.
Bakermans-Kranenburg, M. J., van IJzendoorn, M. H., and Juffer, F. (2003). Less is more: Meta-analyses of sensitivity and attachment interventions in early childhood. *Psychological Bulletin*, 129 (2), 195–215. doi:10.1037/0033-2909.129.2.195

Balint, M. (1937). *Primary Love and Psycho-analytic Technique*. London/New York: Routledge, 2013.

Balint, M. (1968). *The Basic Fault: Therapeutic Aspects of Regression*. London: Tavistock.

Barnard, M., and Barlow, J. (2003). Discovering parental drug dependence: silence and disclosure 1. *Children and Society*, 17(1), 45–56. doi:10.1002/chi.727

Barnett, J. E., Baker, E. K., Elman, N. S., and Schoener, G. R. (2007). In pursuit of wellness: The self-care imperative. *Professional Psychology: Research and Practice*, 38, 603–612.

Bateman, A. and Fonagy, P. (2004). *Psychotherapy for Borderline Personality Disorder. Mentalization Based Treatment*. London: Oxford University Press.

Bateson, G. (1972). *Steps to an Ecology of Mind*. Oxford, UK: Chandler.

Beebe, B. and Lachman, F. (2002). *Infant Research and Adult Treatment*. New York: Analytic Press.

Beebe, B. and Lachmann, F. (2017). *The Mother–Infant Interaction Picture Book: Origins of Attachment*. New York: Norton.

Beebe, B., Lachmann, F. M., and Markese, S. (2012). On the origins of disorganized attachment and internal working models: Paper II. An empirical microanalysis of 4-month mother–infant interaction. *Psychoanalytic Dialogues*, 22 (4), 352–374. doi:10.1080/10481885.2012.679606

Bejerot, N. (1974). *Six Days in August: The Story of the Stockholm Syndrome* (E. King, ed.). New Brunswick, NJ: Rutgers University Press.

Bekir, P., McLellan, T., Childress, A. R., and Gariti, P. (1993). Role reversals in families of substance misusers: A trans-generational phenomenon. *International Journal of the Addictions*, 28(7), 613–630.

Benjamin, J. (1990). *The Bonds of Love: Psychoanalysis, Feminism, and the Problem of Domination*. New York: Pantheon Books.

Benjamin, J. (1995). *Like Subjects, Love Objects: Essays on Recognition and Sexual Difference*. New Haven, CT: Yale University Press.

Benjamin, J. (2018). *Beyond Doer and Done to: Recognition Theory, Intersubjectivity, and the Third*. New York: Routledge.

Bergeret, J. (1974). *La violence fondamentale: Essai de psychopathologie du lien social*. Paris: Dunod.

Bergeret, J. (1981). *Le psychanalyse à l'écoute du toxicomane*. Paris: Dunod.

Berlin, L. J., Zeanah, C. H., and Lieberman, A. F. (2016). Prevention and intervention programs to support early attachment security. In J. Cassidy and P. R. Shaver (eds), *Handbook of Attachment* (3rd edn, pp. 739–758). New York: Guilford.

Bernardi, R., and Eidlin, M. (2018). Thin-skinned or vulnerable narcissism and thick-skinned or grandiose narcissism: Similarities and differences. *The International Journal of Psychoanalysis*, 99 (2), 291–313. doi:10.1080/00207578.2018.1425599

Bion, W. R. (1959). Attacks on linking. *International Journal of Psycho-Analysis*, 40 (5–6),308–315.

Bion, W. R. (1962). A theory of thinking. *International Journal of Psycho-Analysis*, 43, 306–310.

Bion, W. R. (1962). *Learning from Experience*. London: Heinemann.

Bion, W. R. (1963). *Elements of Psycho-analysis*. London: Heinemann.

Bion, W. R. (1965). *Transformations*. London: Heinemann.

Bion, W. R. (1970). *Attention and Interpretation*. London: Karnac.

Bion, W. R. (1974). *Bion's Brazilian Lectures.* London: Karnac, 1990.

Black, K., and Sleigh, M. J. (2013). The impact of parentification on the adjustment of young adults. *Child Psychiatry and Human Development*, 44 (5), 676–688.

Blankstein, J. H. (1970). Gezinstherapie, vanuit psychoanalytisch gezichtspunt. *Tijdschrift voor Psychiatrie*, 12, 186–197.

Boerwinkel, A. R., and Gomperts, W. J. (2001). *Alleen en met z'n tweeën. One- en two-person psychologie in de psychoanalyse.* Assen: Van Gorcum.

Bohm, M. K., and Esser, M. B. (2023). Associations between parental drinking and alcohol use among their adolescent children: findings from a National Survey of United States Parent-Child Dyads. *Journal of Adolescent Health*, 73(5), 961–964. doi:10.1016/j.jadohealth.2023.05.028

Bollas, C. (1987). *The Shadow of the Object: Psychoanalysis of the Unthought Known.* London: Free Association Books.

Bollas, C. (1992). *Being a Character: Psychoanalysis and Self Experience.* New York: Hill and Wang.

Borchet, J., Lewandowska-Walter, A., Połomski, P., Peplinska, A., and Hooper, L. M. (2020). We are in this together: Retrospective parentification, sibling relationships, and self-esteem. *Journal of Child and Family Studies*, 2982–2991. doi:10.1007/s10826–10020–01723–01723

Borossa, J. (1999). Therapeutic relations: Sándor Ferenczi and the British independents. In E. Caldwell (ed.), *Winnicott and the psychoanalytic tradition* (pp. 141–164). London/New York: Routledge, 2018.

Boszormenyi-Nagy, I., and Krasner, B. R. (1986). *Between Give and Take: A Clinical Guide to Contextual Therapy.* New York: Brunner/Mazel.

Boszormenyi-Nagy, I., and Spark, G. M. (1973). *Invisible loyalties: Reciprocity in intergenerational family therapy.* New York: Harper & Row, 1994.

Bourdellon, G. (2004). Engagement dans le désir ou engouffrement dans la dépendance. *Revue Française de Psychanalyse*, LXVIII, 441–457.

Bowen, M. (1978). *Family Therapy in Clinical Practice.* New York: Jason Aronson.

Bowlby, J. (1969). *Attachment and Loss: Vol. 1. Attachment* (2nd edn). New York: Basic Books, 1982.

Bowlby, J. (1973). *Attachment and Loss: Vol. 2. Separation: Anxiety and Anger.* New York: Basic Books.

Bowlby, J. (1977). The making and breaking of affectional bonds: II. Some principles of psychotherapy: The Fiftieth Maudsley Lecture (expanded version). *The British Journal of Psychiatry*, 130(5), 421–431. doi:10.1192/bjp.130.5.421

Bowlby, J. (1980). *Attachment and Loss: Vol. 3. Loss: Sadness and Depression.* New York: Basic Books.

Bowlby, J. (1988). *A Secure Base. Clinical Applications of Attachment Theory.* London/New York: Routledge.

Braunstein, N. (1992). *La jouissance. Un concept Lacanien.* Paris: Point hors ligne.

Bregman, R. (2024). *Moral Ambition: Stop Wasting Your Talent and Start Making a Difference.* New York: Bloomsbury.

Bromberg, P. M. (2011). *The Shadow of the Tsunami and the Growth of the Relational Mind.* New York: Routledge.

Bucci, W. (1999). *Psychoanalysis and Cognitive Science: A Multiple Code Theory.* New York: Guilford Press.

Burnett, G., Jones, R. A., Bliwise, N. G., and Ross, L. T. (2006). *Family unpredictability, parental alcoholism, and the development of parentification. American Journal of Family Therapy*, 34 (3), 181–189. doi:10.1080/01926180600550437

Burton, L. (2007). Childhood adultification in economically disadvantaged families: A conceptual model. *Family Relations*, 56 (4), 329–345. doi:10.1111/ j.1741–3729.2007.00463.x

Byng-Hall, J. (1995). Creating a secure family base: Some implications of attachment theory for family therapy. *Family Process*, 34 (1), 45–58. doi:10.1111/j.1545-5300.1995.00045.x

Byng-Hall J. (1995). *Rewriting Family Scripts*. New York: Guilford.

Byng-Hall, J. (2002). Relieving parentified children's burdens in families with insecure attachment patterns. *Family Process*. 41 (3), 375–388. doi:10.1111/j.1545-5300.2002.41307.x

Byng-Hall, J. (2008). The significance of children fulfilling parental roles: Implications for family therapy. *Journal of Family Therapy*, 30 (2), 147–162. doi:10.1111/j.1467–6427.2008.00423.x

Cain, N. R. (2000). Psychotherapists with personal histories of psychiatric hospitalization. *Psychiatric Rehabilitation Journal*, 24, 22–28. https://psycnet.apa.org/doi/10.1037/h0095127

Cambien, J. (1988). Fantasie in het werk van Melanie Klein. *Tijdschrift voor Psychotherapie*, 14, 258–268.

Champion, J. E., Jaser, S. S., Reeslund, K. L., Simmons, L., Potts, J. E., Shears, A. R., and Compas, B. E. (2009). Caretaking behaviors by adolescent children of mothers with and without a history of depression. *Journal of Family Psychology*, 23 (2), 156–166. doi:10.1037/a0014978

Chase, N. D. (1999). Parentification: An overview of theory, research and societal issues. In: N. D. Chase (ed.), *Burdened Children: Theory, Research and Treatment of Parentification*. Thousand Oaks, CA: Sage.

Chase, N. D., Deming, M. P. and Wells, M. C. (1998). Parentification, parental alcoholism, and academic status among young adults, *American Journal of Family Therapy*, 26, 105–114. doi:10.1080/01926189808251091

Chemla, P. (2009). Neutralité malveillante. *La Clinique lacanienne*, 15, 43–59.

Chen, C.-Y.-C., and Panebianco, A. (2019). Physical and psychological conditions of parental chronic illness, parentification and adolescent psychological adjustment. *Psychology and Health*, 35 (9), 1075–1094. doi:10.1080/ 08870446.2019.1699091

Cho, A. R., and Lee, S. Y. (2019). Exploring effects of childhood parentification on adult-depressive symptoms in Korean college students. *Journal of Clinical Psychology*, 75 (4), 801–813. doi:10.1002/jclp.22737

Cicchetti, D. and Toth, S. (1995). Developmental psychopathology perspective on child abuse and neglect. *Journal of the American Academy of Child and Adolescent Psychiatry*1995; 34 (5), 541–565.

Clark, E. L., Jiao, Y., Sandoval, K., and Biringen, Z. (2021). Neurobiological implications of parent–child emotional availability: A review. *Brain Sciences*, 11 (8), 1016. doi:10.3390/brainsci11081016

Cleaver, H., Unell, I., and Aldgate, J. (2011). *Children's Needs–Parenting Capacity: Child Abuse, Parental Mental Illness, Learning Disability, Substance Misuse and Domestic Violence* (2nd edn). London: The Stationery Office.

Conchar, C., and Repper, J. (2014). 'Walking wounded or wounded healer?' Does personal experience of mental health problems help or hinder mental health practice? A review of the literature. *Mental Health and Social Inclusion*, 18, 35–44. doi:10.1108/MHSI-02-2014-0003

Crittenden, P. M. (2017). *Raising Parents: Attachment, Representation, and Treatment*, London/New York: Routledge.

Cuijpers, P. and Bolier L. (2001). *Drankjewel: Een zelfhulpgids voor volwassen kinderen van probleemdrinkers.* Utrecht: Trimbos-Instituut.

Cuijpers P., Langendoen, Y. and Bijl R. V. (1999). Psychiatric disorders in adult children of problem drinkers: prevalence, first onset and comparison with other risk factors. *Addiction*, 94 (10), 1489–1498. doi:10.1046/j.1360-0443.1999.941014895.x

Dariotis, J. K., Lorenzo, K., Turkheimer, E., Perlstein, M. B., and White, C. N. (2023). Parentification: Vulnerability, reactivity, resilience, and thriving—A mixed-methods systematic literature review. *Adversity and Resilience Science*, 4 (2), 127–166.

Dayton, T. (2000). *Trauma and Addiction: Ending the Cycle of Pain through Emotional Literacy.* Deerfield Beach, FL: Health Communication Inc.

De Cauter, L (2011). *De Oorsprongen of het Boek der Verbazing*. Leuven: LannooCampus.

de Gaulejac, V. (1987). *La névrose de classe: trajectoire sociale et conflits d'identité.* Paris: Hommes et Groupes éditeurs.

De Kloet, E. R. (2009). Stress: neurobiologisch perspectief. *Tijdschrift voor Psychiatrie*, 51 (8), 541–550.

De Vleminck, J. (2023). Ferenczi met Winnicott over het infantiele trauma. In: Franckx, C. and Hebbrecht, M. *Het kinderlijk trauma. Verloren tussen tederheid en passie* (pp. 221–237). Antwerpen/'s-Hertogenbosch: Gompel and Svacina.

De Vries, A., and Eskens, E. (2017). *Amor fati: Filosoferen tegen het einde – brieven van en voor een stervende filosoof.* Zaltbommel, NL: Vrije Uitgevers.

De Wolf, M. H. M. (2015). *Psychoanalytische theorievorming en de DSM-5*. Bussum: Coutinho.

Dickeson, E., Mazerolle, S. M., and Pitney, W. A. (2017). The prevalence and implications of wounded healers: A systematic review of the literature. *Athletic Training Education Journal*, 12 (4), 276–286. doi:10.4085/1204276

Dolto, F. (1988). *Quand les parents se séparent* (I. de Angelino, coauthor.). Paris: Seuil.

Domenico, D., and Windle, M. (1993). Parental alcoholism and adult female offspring: Negative life events, personal resources, depression, and parenting. *Journal of Marriage and the Family*, 55 (2), 325–335.

Donnay-Richelle, J., Timsit, M. and Dongier, M. (1972). Study of the deep motivations of vocational choice in psychiatry candidates and students in psychology. *Acta Psychiatrica Belgica*, 72, 345–346.

Duchamp, M. (1957). The creative act. In: A. Sanouillet and E. Peterson (eds), *The Writings of Marcel Duchamp*. New York: Da Capo Press, 1973.

Duffy, R. D., and Dik, B. J. (2013). *Make Your Job a Calling: How the Psychology of Vocation Can Change Your Life at Work*. West Conshohocken: Templeton Press.

Durant, W. (1926). *The Story of Philosophy: The Lives and Opinions of the World's Greatest Philosophers.* New York: Simon and Schuster, 2012.

Eco, U. (1962). *The Open Work*, translated by Anna Cancogni with an Introduction by David Robey. Cambridge, MA: Harvard UP, 1989.

El-Guebaly, N., Offord, D. R., and Boyle, M. H. (1993). Individual and familial characteristics of children of alcoholics. *The Canadian Journal of Psychiatry*, 38 (7), 472–480.

Elkind, D. (1981). *The Hurried Child: Growing Up Too Fast Too Soon* (3rd edn). Cambridge, MA: Da Capo Press, 2007.

Engelhardt, J. A. (2012). The developmental implications of parentification: Effects on childhood attachment. *Graduate Student Journal of Psychology*, 14, 45–52.

Etchegoyen, H., Lopez, B. and Rabih, M. (1987), Envy and how to interpret it. *International Journal of Psycho-Analysis*, 68, 49–61.

Fagan, B. M., and Durrani, N. (1971). *People of the Earth: An Introduction to World Prehistory.* London/New York: Routledge, 2016.

Fairbairn, W. R. D. (1943). The repression and the return of bad objects. *Psycho-analytic Studies of the Personality* (pp. 59–81). London: Tavistock, 1952.

Farber, B. A., Manevich, I., Metzger, J., and Saypol, E. (2005). Choosing psychotherapy as a career: Why did we cross that road? *Journal of Clinical Psychology*, 61, 1009–1031. doi:10.1002/jclp.20174

Fenichel, O. (1946). *The Psychoanalytic Theory of the Neuroses.* New York: Norton.

Ferenchick, E., and Rosenthal, D. (2019). Identified patient in family systems theory. In J. Lebow, A. Chambers, and D. C. Breunlin (eds), *Encyclopedia of Couple and Family Therapy* (pp. 1431–1433). Cham: Springer.

Ferenczi, S. (1927). Die Anpassung der Familie an das Kind. *Bausteine zur Psycho-analyse, Band III: Arbeiten aus den Jahren 1908–1933* (pp. 347–366). Bern/Stuttgart: Hans Huber, 1964.

Ferenczi, S. (1928). Die Elastizität der psychoanalytischen Technik. *Bausteine zur Psychoanalyse, Band III: Arbeiten aus den Jahren 1908–1933* (pp. 380–398). Bern/Stuttgart: Hans Huber, 1964.

Ferenczi, S. (1928). The elasticity of psycho-analytic technique. In M. Balint (ed.), *Final Contributions to the Problems and Methods of Psycho-Analysis* (pp. 87–101). London: Hogarth, 1955.

Ferenczi, S. (1930). Relaxationsprinzip und Neokatharsis. *Bausteine zur Psycho-analyse, Band III: Arbeiten aus den Jahren 1908–1933* (pp. 468–489). Bern/Stuttgart: Hans Huber, 1964.

Ferenczi, S. (1931). Kinderanalysen mit Erwachsenen. *Bausteine zur Psychoanalyse, Band III: Arbeiten aus den Jahren 1908–1933* (pp. 490–510). Bern/Stuttgart: Hans Huber, 1964.

Ferenczi, S. (1932). *The Clinical Diary of Sándor Ferenczi* (M. Balint, ed.; M. Dupont, trans.). Cambridge, MA: Harvard University Press, 1988.

Fernando, J. (2009). *The Processes of Defence: Trauma, Drives, and Reality—A New Synthesis.* London: Karnac.

Ferro, A. (2002). Narrative derivatives of the analytic field. *International Journal of Psycho-Analysis*, 83 (4), 807–818.

Finell, J. S. (1985). Narcissistic problems in analysts. *International Journal of Psycho-analytic Psychotherapy*, 9, 227–231.

Fink, B. (1995). *The Lacanian Subject: Between Language and Jouissance.* Princeton, NJ: Princeton University Press.

Fischer, J. L., and Crawford, D. W. (1992). Codependence and parenting styles. *Family Relations*, 41 (2), 204–210.

Fonagy, P., and Campbell, C. (2019). Mentalizing, attachment and epistemic trust: how psychotherapy can promote resilience. *Journal of Child Psychotherapy*, 45 (1), 91–108. https://discovery.ucl.ac.uk/id/eprint/1574378.

Fonagy, P., and Target, M. (2003). *Psychoanalytic Theories: Perspectives from Developmental Psychopathology*. London: Whurr.

Fonagy, P., Gergely, G., Jurist, E., and Target, M. (2002). *Affect Regulation, Mentalization, and the Development of the Self.* New York: Other Press.

Fonagy, P., Luyten, P., and Allison, E. (2015). Epistemic petrification and the restoration of epistemic trust: a new conceptualization of borderline personality disorder and its treatment. *Journal of Personality Disorders*, 29 (5), 575–609. doi:10.1521/pedi.2015.29.5.575

Fonagy, P., Steele, M., Steele, H., Higgitt, A. and Target, M. (1994). The theory and practice of resilience. *Journal of Child Psychology and Psychiatry*, 15, 231–257. doi:10.1111/j.1469-7610.1994.tb01160.x

Fonagy, P., Steele, M., Steele, H., Moran, G. S., and Higgitt, A. C. (1991). The capacity for understanding mental states: The reflective self in parent and child and its significance for security of attachment. *Infant Mental Health Journal*, 12 (3), 201–218. doi:10.1002/1097-0355(199123)12:3

Fraiberg, S., Adelson, E., and Shapiro, V. (1975). Ghosts in the nursery: A psychoanalytic approach to the problems of impaired mother–infant relationships. *Journal of the American Academy of Child Psychiatry*, 14 (3), 387–421. doi:10.1016/S0002-7138(09)61442–61444

Franckx, C. and Hebbrecht, M. (eds) (2023). *Het kinderlijk trauma. Verloren tussen tederheid en passie.* Antwerpen; 's-Hertogenbosch: Gompel and Svacina.

Freud, A. (1927). Four lectures on child analysis. In *The Writings of Anna Freud* (Vol. I). New York: International Universities Press, 1974.

Freud, A. (1936). The Ego and the Mechanisms of Defence. In *The Writings of Anna Freud* (Vol. II, pp. 3–191). New York: International Universities Press, 1974.

Freud, A. (1936). *The Ego and the Mechanisms of Defence. The Writings of Anna Freud (Vol. II)*. New York: International Universities Press, 1974.

Freud, S. (1895). *Het ontwerp* (G. Van de Vijver and F. Geerardyn, vert. and inl.). Gent, België: Idesça, 1992.

Freud, S. (1900). *The Interpretation of Dreams* (J. Strachey, trans.). New York: Basic Books, 1953.

Freud, S. (1905). Three essays on the theory of sexuality. In J. Strachey (ed. and trans.), *S. E.* (Vol. 7, pp. 125–245). London: Hogarth, 1953.

Freud, S. (1908). Character and anal erotism. In *S. E.* (Vol. 9, pp. 167–175). London: Hogarth.

Freud, S. (1909). De familieroman van de neuroticus. In *Werken* (Vol. 4, pp. 547–550). Amsterdam: Boom, 2006.

Freud, S. (1910). A special type of choice of object made by men (Contributions to the psychology of love I). In *S. E.* (Vol. 11, pp. 165–175). London: Hogarth.

Freud, S. (1910). 'Wild' psycho-analysis. In *S. E.* (Vol. 11, pp. 219–227). London: Hogarth, 1957.

Freud, S. (1912). Recommendations to physicians practising psycho-analysis. In *S. E.* (Vol. 12, pp. 109–120). London: Hogarth, 1958.

Freud, S. (1914). On narcissism: An introduction. In *S. E.* (Vol. 14, pp. 73–102). London: Hogarth, 1957.

Freud, S. (1914). Remembering, repeating and working-through. In *S. E.* (Vol. 12, pp. 145–156). London: Hogarth, 1958.

Freud, S. (1915). Driften en hun lotgevallen. In *Werken* (Vol. 7, pp. 17–44). Amsterdam: Boom, 2006.
Freud, S. (1915). Instincts and their vicissitudes. In *S. E.* (Vol. 14, pp. 109–140). London: Hogarth.
Freud, S. (1915). Repression. In *S. E.* (Vol. 14, pp. 143–158). London: Hogarth.
Freud, S. (1915). The unconscious. In *S. E.* (Vol. 14, pp. 159–215). London: Hogarth, 1961.
Freud, S. (1916–1917). Colleges inleiding tot de psychoanalyse. In *Werken* (Vol. 7, pp. 211–613). Amsterdam: Boom, 2006.
Freud, S. (1917). Introductory lectures on psycho-analysis (Part III). In *S.E.* (Vol. 16, pp. 243–463). London: Hogarth, 1963.
Freud, S. (1920). Aan gene zijde van het lustprincipe. In *Psychoanalytische theorie* (Vol. 1). Amsterdam: Boom.
Freud, S. (1920). Beyond the pleasure principle. In *S. E.* (Vol. 18, pp. 1–64). London: Hogarth, 1961.
Freud, S. (1921). Group psychology and the analysis of the ego. In *S. E.* (Vol. 18, pp. 65–143). London: Hogarth, 1955.
Freud, S. (1923). The ego and the id. In *S. E.* (Vol. 19, pp. 12–66). London: Hogarth, 1961.
Freud, S. (1926). The question of lay analysis. In *S. E.* (Vol. 20, pp. 179–258). London: Hogarth, 1969.
Freud, S. (1930). Civilization and its discontents. In *S. E.* (Vol. 21, pp. 57–145). London: Hogarth, 1961.
Freud, S. (1933). Colleges inleiding tot de psychoanalyse – Nieuwe reeks. In *Werken* (Vol. 10, pp. 79–232). Amsterdam: Boom, 2006.
Freud, S. (1937). Analysis terminable and interminable. In *S. E.* (Vol. 23, pp. 209–254). London: Hogarth, 1964.
Freud, S. (1937). Constructions in analysis. In *S. E.* (Vol. 23, pp. 255–270). London: Hogarth, 1964.
Freud, S., and Ferenczi, S. (1996). *The Correspondence of Sigmund Freud and Sándor Ferenczi* (E. Falzeder, E. Brabant, and P. Giampieri-Deutsch, eds). Cambridge, MA/London: The Belknap Press of Harvard University Press.
Fussell, F. W., and Bonney, W. C. (1990). A comparative study of childhood experiences of psychotherapists and physicists: Implications for clinical practice. *Psychotherapy: Theory, Research, Practice, Training*, 27 (4), 505–512.
Gabbard, G. O. (1995). When the patient is a therapist. Special challenges in the psychoanalysis of mental health professionals. *Psychoanalytic Review*, 82, pp. 709–725.
Gabbard, G. O. (2000). On gratitude and gratification. *Journal of the American Psychoanalytic Association*, 48 (3), 698–716.
Gabbard, G. O. (2014). *Psychodynamic Psychiatry in Clinical Practice* (5th edn). Washington, DC: American Psychiatric Publishing.
Gabbard, G. O., and Wilkinson, S. M. (2000). *Management of Countertransference with Borderline Patients*. Plymouth, UK: Rowman and Littlefield Publishers, Inc.
Garber, B. D. (2011). Parental alienation and the dynamics of the enmeshed parent–child dyad: Adultification, parentification, and infantilization. *Family Court Review*, 49 (2), 322–335. doi:10.1111/j.1744-1617.2011.01374.x
Gilford, T. T., and Reynolds, A. (2011). 'My mother's keeper': The effects of parentification on black female college students. *Journal of Black Psychology*, 37 (1), 55–77. doi:10.1177/0095798410372624.

Glover, E. (1932). On the etiology of drug addiction. *On the Early Development of the Mind* (pp. 187–215). London: Imago, 1956.

Goethe, J.W. (1832). 'Faust – Deel Twee'. In: J.W. von Goethe (1982). *Faust*. Deel Een en Twee. Amsterdam: Wereldbibliotheek.

Goglia, L. R., Jurkovic, G. J., Burt, A. M., and Burge-Callaway, K. G. (1992). Generational boundary distortions by adult children of alcoholics: Child-as-parent and child-as-mate. *The American Journal of Family Therapy* 20 (4), 291–299. doi:10.1080/01926189208250899

Goldner, L., Jakobi, C. D., Schorr, S., Dakak, S., and Shawahne, N. (2021). Keep it quiet: Mother–daughter parentification and difficulties in separation–individuation shaping daughters' authentic/true self and self-silencing: A mediation model. *Psychoanalytic Psychology*, 39 (2), 165–174. doi:10.1037/pap0000352

Goldner, L., Sachar, S. C., and Abir, A. (2019). Mother-adolescent parentification, enmeshment and adolescents' intimacy: The mediating role of rejection sensitivity. *Journal of Child and Family Studies*, 28 (1), 192–201. doi:10.1007/ s10826–10018–1244–1248

Green, A. (1995). *La causalité psychique. Entre nature et culture*. Paris: Odile Jacob.

Grotstein, J. (1981). Who is the dreamer who dreams the dream and who is the dreamer who understands it?*Do I Dare Disturb the Universe?* (pp. 110–145). London: Karnac.

Hebbrecht, M. (2023). Het klinische dagboek van Sándor Ferenczi. Psychoanalyse van trauma. In Franckx, C. and Hebbrecht, M., *Het kinderlijk trauma. Verloren tussen tederheid en passie* (pp. 157–170). Antwerpen/'s Hertogenbosch: Gompel and Svacina.

Hegel, G. W. F. (1830). *The Philosophy of History* (J. Sibree, trans.). New York: Dover, 1956.

Heraclitus. (1987). *Fragments: A Text and Translation* (T. M. Robinson, ed. and trans.). Toronto: University of Toronto Press.

Hesse, E. (2008). The Adult Attachment Interview: Protocol, method of analysis, and empirical studies. In J. Cassidy and P. R. Shaver (eds), *Handbook of Attachment: Theory, Research, and Clinical Applications* (2nd edn, pp. 552–598). New York: Guilford.

Hetherington, E. M. (1999). Should we stay together for the sake of the children? In E. M. Hetherington (ed.), *Coping with Divorce, Single Parenting, and Remarriage: A Risk and Resiliency Perspective* (pp. 93–116). New York: Lawrence Erlbaum.

Hicks, H. R. (2023) Experiences and long-term implications of childhood parentification and parental substance misuse: a scoping review, *McNair Scholars Research Journal*, 26, Article 6. doi:10.32855/2642-2492.1005

Hicks, S. (Director). (1996). *Shine* [Film]. Momentum Pictures.

Hinshelwood, R. D. (1991). *A Dictionary of Kleinian Thought*. London: Free Association Books.

Holt, A. (2015). *Working with Adolescent Violence and Abuse Towards Parents: Approaches and Contexts for Intervention*. London/New York: Routledge.

Holzer, J. (1983–1985). Protect Me from What I Want. LED Sign. *Survival Series*.

Hooper, L. M. (2008) Defining and understanding parentification. *The Alabama Counseling Association Journal* 34 (1), 34–43.

Hooper, L. M., and Doehler, K. (2012). Assessing family caregiving: A comparison of three retrospective parentification measures. *Journal of Marital and Family Therapy*, 38 (4), 653–666. doi:10.1111/j.1752-0606.2011.00258.x

Hooper, L. M., and Wallace, S. A. (2010). Evaluating the parentification questionnaire: Psychometric properties and psychopathology correlates. *Contemporary Family Therapy*, 32 (1), 52–68. doi:10.1007/s10591-009-9103-9

Hooper, L. M., DeCoster, J., White, N., and Voltz, M. L. (2011). Characterizing the magnitude of the relation between self-reported childhood parentification and adult psychopathology: A meta-analysis. *Journal of Clinical Psychology*, 67 (10), 1028–1043. doi:10.1002/jclp.20807

Hope, A., Barry, J., and Byrne, S. (2018). *The Untold Story: Harms Experienced in the Irish Population Due to Others' Drinking*. Dublin: Health Service Executive (HSE).

Hoste, M. (2010) Verslaving: de ideale voedingsbodem voor parentificatie. In: M. Kinet (ed.) *Parentificatie. Als het kind te snel ouder wordt* (pp. 123–146). Antwerpen/Apeldoorn: Garant.

Hyysalo, N., Gastelle, M., and Flykt, M. (2022). Maternal pre-and postnatal substance use and attachment in young children: A systematic review and meta-analysis. *Development and Psychopathology*, 34 (4), 1231–1248. doi:10.1017/S0954579421000134

Jackson, D. D. (1965). The study of the family. *Family Process*, 4 (1), 1–20.

Jackson, E. F., Raval, V. V., Bendikas-King, E. A., Raval, P. H., and Trivedi, S. S. (2016). Cultural variation in reports of subjective experience of parent-child boundary dissolution among emerging adults. *Journal of Family Issues*, 37 (5), 671–691. doi:10.1177/0192513X15576280

Johnson, S. M. (2019). *Attachment Theory in Practice: Emotionally Focused Therapy (EFT) with Individuals, Couples, and Families*. New York: Guilford.

Jung, C. G. (1951). *Memories, Dreams, Reflections* (A. Jaffé, ed.; R. Winston and C. Winston, trans.). New York: Vintage, 1983.

Jurkovic, G. J. (1997). *Lost Childhoods: The Plight of the Parentified Child*. New York: Brunner/Mazel, 2014.

Jurkovic, G. J., Morrell, R., and Thirkield, A. (1999). Assessing parentification: guidelines for researchers and clinicians. In: N. D. Chase (ed.), *Burdened Children: Theory, Research and Treatment of Parentification*. London, New Delhi: Sage Publications, 93–96.

Kane, K., Westman, J., Gissler, M., Jayaram-Lindström, N., and Franck, J. (2024). Risk of severe mood and anxiety disorders in the adult children of parents with alcohol use disorder: A nationwide cohort study. *Journal of Epidemiology and Community Health*, 78 (7), 444–452. doi:10.1136/jech-2023-221720

Kelley, M. L., French, A., Bountress, K., Keefe, H. A., Schroeder, V., Steer, K., Fals-Stewart, W., and Gumienny, L. (2007). Parentification and family responsibility in the family of origin of adult children of alcoholics. *Addictive Behaviors*, 32 (4), 675–685. doi:10.1016/j.addbeh.2006.06.010

Kennedy, B. S., and Black, T. G. (2010). Life outside the 50-minute hour: The personal lives of counsellors. *Canadian Journal of Counselling and Psychotherapy*, 44, 421–437. https://cjc-rcc.ucalgary.ca/article/view/59243

Kerig, P. K. (2005). Revisiting the construct of boundary dissolution: A multidimensional perspective. *Journal of Emotional Abuse*, 1, 5–42. doi:10.4324/9781315821085–7

Kernberg, O. F. (1975). *Borderline Conditions and Pathological Narcissism*. New York: Jason Aronson.

Kernberg, O. F. (1984). *Severe Personality Disorders: Psychotherapeutic Strategies.* New Haven, CT: Yale University Press.

Kernberg, O. F. (2004). *Aggression in Personality Disorders and Perversions.* New Haven, CT: Yale University Press.

Kernberg, O. F., Yeomans, F. E., Clarkin, J. F., and Levy, K. N. (2008). Transference focused psychotherapy: Overview and update. *International Journal of Psychoanalysis,* 89 (3), 601–620. doi:10.1111/j.1745-8315.2008.00046.x

Kets de Vries, M. (2010). *Leadership Coaching and the Rescuer Syndrome: How to Manage Both Sides of the Couch.* Faculty and Research and Working Paper. Geneve: INSEAD.

Kinet, M. (1996). Weerzien met…Melanie Klein. *Tijdschrift voor Psychotherapie,* 22, 197–211.

Kinet, M. (2006) Een langgerekte kortsluiting. *Zuchtigheid en afhankelijkheid* (pp. 9–23). Antwerpen-Apeldoorn: Garant.

Kinet, M. (2006). *Freud & Co in de psychiatrie. Klinisch-psychotherapeutisch perspectief.* Antwerpen/Apeldoorn: Garant.

Kinet, M. (2008) (ed.) *Psychoanalyse en/van het Systeem. Bij jongeren en hun gezin.* Antwerpen/Apeldoorn: Garant.

Kinet, M. (ed.) (2010). *Parentificatie. Als het kind te snel ouder wordt.* Antwerpen/Apeldoorn: Garant.

Kinet, M. (2019). Enkele oedipale variaties. Van Darwin tot Lacan. In Kinet, M., and Heuves, W. (eds), *Driehoeksverhoudingen. Actuele oedipale variaties* (pp. 51–70). Antwerpen/'s-Hertogenbosch: Gompel and Svacina.

Kinet, M. (2023). *The Spirit of the Drive in Neuropsychoanalysis.* London/New York: Routledge.

Kinet, M. (2023). Tussen ça voir en faire ainsi. In Franckx, C. and Hebbrecht, M., *Het kinderlijk trauma. Verloren tussen tederheid en passie* (pp. 293–305). Antwerpen/'s-Hertogenbosch: Gompel and Svacina.

Kinet, M. (2024). *Psychoanalytic Principles in Psychiatric Practice. A Remedy by Truth.* London/New York: Routledge.

Kinet, M. (2025). *Psychoanalytic Psychotherapy in Psychiatric Practice. Premises and Clinical Portraits.* London/New York: Routledge.

Kinet, M. (2025). *Patient Testimonies of Psychodynamic Psychotherapy. Reported and Recorded.* London/New York: Routledge.

Kinet, M. (2025). Che Vuoi? Epiloog in enkele contrapunten. In Hebbrecht, M. and De Vleminck, J. (eds) *Verleiding en vertaling. Het enigma van de seksualiteit* (pp. 173–189). Antwerpen/'s-Hertogenbosch: Gompel and Svacina.

Kinet, M. and Vermote, R. (eds) (2005). *Mentalisatie.* Antwerpen/Apeldoorn: Garant.

Klasen, J., Nolte, T., Möller, H., and Taubner, S. (2019). Aversive Kindheitserfahrungen, Bindungsrepräsentationen und Mentalisierungsfähigkeit von Psychotherapeuten in Ausbildung. *Zeitschrift für Psychosomatische Medizin und Psychotherapie,* 65 (4). doi:10.13109/zptm.2019.65.4.353

Klein, M. (1935). A contribution to the psychogenesis of manic-depressive states. *Love, Guilt and Reparation and Other Works 1921–1945* (pp. 262–289). London: Hogarth, 1975.

Klein, M. (1937). Love, guilt and reparation. In *Love, Guilt and Reparation and Other Works 1921–1945* (pp. 306–343). London: Virago, 1988.

Klein, M. (1940). Mourning and its relation to manic-depressive states. *Love, Guilt and Reparation and Other Works 1921–1945* (pp. 344–369). London: Virago, 1988.

Klein, M. (1946). Notes on some schizoid mechanisms. *Envy and Gratitude and Other Works 1946–1963* (pp. 1–24). London: Hogarth, 1975.

Klein, M. (1955). The psycho-analytic play technique: Its history and significance. In *Envy and Gratitude and Other Works 1946–1963* (pp. 122–140). London: Virago, 1988.

Klein, M. (1957). Envy and gratitude. In *Envy and Gratitude and Other Works 1946–1963* (pp. 176–235). London: Virago, 1988.

Klein, M. (1959). Our adult world and its roots in infancy. In *Envy and gratitude and other works 1946–1963* (pp. 247–263). London: Virago, 1988.

Kohut, H. (1971). *The Analysis of the Self.* New York: International Universities Press.

Kohut, H. (1977). *The Restoration of the Self.* New York: International Universities Press.

Koob, G. F., and Volkow, N. D. (2016). Neurobiology of addiction: A neurocircuitry analysis. *The Lancet Psychiatry*, 3 (8), 760–773. doi:10.1016/S2215-0366(16)00104-00108

Kornaszewska-Polak, M. (2019). Attachment in adult children of alcoholics. *Current Issues in Personality Psychology*, 7 (1), 1–12.

Kreisman, J. J., and Straus, H. (1989). *I Hate You, Don't Leave Me: Understanding the Borderline Personality.* New York: Avon.

Kundakovic, M., and Champagne, F. A. (2014). Early-life experience, epigenetics, and the developing brain. *Neuropsychopharmacology*, 39 (1), 244–256. doi:10.1038/npp.2013.1559

Kuppens, S., Moore, S. C., Gross, V., Lowthian, E., and Siddaway, A. P. (2020). The enduring effects of parental alcohol, tobacco, and drug use on child well-being: A multilevel meta-analysis. *Development and psychopathology*, 32 (2), 765–778. doi:10.1017/S0954579419000749

Lacan, J. (1949). Le stade du miroir comme formateur de la fonction du Je. *Écrits* (pp. 93–100). Paris: Seuil, 1966.

Lacan, J. (1953). Fonction et champ de la parole et du langage en psychanalyse. *Écrits* (pp. 237–322). Paris: Seuil, 1966.

Lacan, J. (1953–1954). *Le Séminaire, Livre I: Les écrits techniques de Freud* (J.-A. Miller, ed.). Paris: Seuil, 1975.

Lacan, J. (1954–1955). *Le Séminaire, Livre II: Le moi dans la théorie de Freud et dans la technique de la psychanalyse* (J.-A. Miller, ed.). Paris: Seuil, 1978.

Lacan, J. (1955). La chose freudienne ou Sens du retour à Freud en psychanalyse. *Écrits* (pp. 401–436). Paris: Seuil, 1966.

Lacan, J. (1955). Variantes de la cure-type. *Écrits* (pp. 323–349). Paris: Seuil, 1966.

Lacan, J. (1956–1957). *Le Séminaire, Livre IV: La relation d'objet* (J.-A. Miller, ed.). Paris: Seuil, 1994.

Lacan, J. (1957–1958). *Le Séminaire, Livre V: Les formations de l'inconscient* (J.-A. Miller, ed.). Paris: Seuil, 1998.

Lacan, J. (1959–1960). *Le Séminaire, Livre VII: L'éthique de la psychanalyse* (J.-A. Miller, ed.). Paris: Seuil, 1986.

Lacan, J. (1959–1960). *The Seminar of Jacques Lacan, Book VII: The Ethics of Psychoanalysis, 1959–1960* (D. Porter, trans.). New York: Norton, 1992.

Lacan, J. (1962–1963). *Le Séminaire, Livre X: L'angoisse* (J.-A. Miller, ed.). Paris: Seuil, 2004.

Lacan, J. (1964). *Le Séminaire, Livre XI: Les quatre concepts fondamentaux de la psychanalyse* (J.-A. Miller, ed.). Paris: Seuil.

Lacan, J. (1964). *The Four Fundamental Concepts of Psycho-analysis* (A. Sheridan, trans.). New York: Norton, 1977.

Lacan, J. (1966). *Écrits.* Paris: Seuil.

Lacan, J. (1966). *Écrits: A selection* (A. Sheridan, trans.). London: Tavistock, 1977.

Lacan, J. (1966–1967). *Le Séminaire, Livre XIV: La logique du fantasme* (J.-A. Miller, ed.). Paris: Seuil, 2023.

Lacan, J. (1991). *The Seminar of Jacques Lacan, Book V: The Formations of the Unconscious* (J.-A. Miller, ed.). Cambridge: Polity Press.

Lacan, J. (2005). *Le Séminaire, Livre XXIV: L'insu que sait de l'une-bévue s'aile à mourre (1976–1977)* (J.-A. Miller, ed.). Paris: Seuil.

Lamia, M. C. and Krieger, M. J. (2015). *The White Knight Syndrome. Rescuing Yourself from Your Need to Rescue Others.* Brattleboro: Echo Point Books.

Lampe, P. (2002). *Het Moeder Theresasyndroom, het persoonlijke motief in de hulpverlening*. Amsterdam: Boom.

Laplanche, J., and Pontalis, J.-B. (1973). *The Language of Psycho-analysis* (D. Nicholson-Smith, trans.). New York: Norton.

Laverdière, O., Kealy, D., Ogrodniczuk, J. S., Chamberland, S., and Descôteaux, J. (2019). Psychotherapists' professional quality of life. *Traumatology*, 25, 208–215.

Lemma, A. (2015). *Introduction to the Practice of Psychoanalytic Psychotherapy.* New York: Wiley.

Levy, K. N., Meehan, K. B., Kelly, K. M., Reynoso, J. S., Weber, M., Clarkin, J. F., and Kernberg, O. F. (2006). Change in attachment patterns and reflective function in a randomized control trial of transference-focused psychotherapy for borderline personality disorder. *Journal of Consulting and Clinical Psychology*, 74 (6), 1027–1040.

Lieberman, A. F., Ghosh Ippen, C., and Van Horn, P. (2015). Infant–parent psychotherapy: An evidence-based treatment for early trauma. In J. D. Osofsky (ed.), *Handbook of Infant Mental Health* (3rd edn, pp. 439–449). New York: Guilford.

Lieberman, A. F., Padrón, E., Van Horn, P., and Harris, W. W. (2005). Angels in the nursery: The intergenerational transmission of benevolent parental influences. *Infant Mental Health Journal*, 26 (6), 504–520. doi:10.1002/imhj.20071

Lingiardi, V., and McWilliams, N. (2018). Introduction to the special issue on the Psychodynamic Diagnostic Manual, (PDM-2): The PDM: Yesterday, today, tomorrow. *Psychoanalytic Psychology*, 35 (3), 289. doi:10.1037/pap0000188

Loach, K. (Director). (2019). *Sorry We Missed You* [Film]. Sixteen Films; Why Not Productions; Wild Bunch.

Loose, R. (2002). *The Subject of Addiction. Psychoanalysis and the Administration of Enjoyment*. London/New York: Karnac.

Love, P. and Robinson, P. (1990). *The Emotional Incest Syndrome: What to Do When a Parent's Love Rules Your Life.* New York: Bantam.

Luborsky, L., Crits-Christoph, P., McLellan, A. T., Woody, G., Piper, W., Liberman, B., Imber, S., and Pilkonis, P. (1986). Do therapists vary much in their success? Findings from four outcome studies. *American Journal of Orthopsychiatry*, 56 (4), 501–512.

Luyten, P., and Fonagy, P. (2015). The neurobiology of mentalizing. *Personality Disorders: Theory, Research, and Treatment*, 6 (4), 366–379. doi:10.1037/per0000117

Lyons-Ruth, K. (1998). Implicit relational knowing: its role in development and psychoanalytic treatment. *Infant Mental Health Journal*, 19, 282–289.

Lyons-Ruth, K. (2002). Dissociation and the parent-infant dialogue: a longitudinal perspective from attachment research. *Journal of the American Psychoanalytical Association*, 51 (3), 884–911.

Lyons-Ruth, K., and Jacobvitz, D. (1999). Attachment disorganization: Unresolved loss, relational violence, and lapses in behavioral and attentional strategies. In J. Cassidy and P. R. Shaver (eds), *Handbook of Attachment: Theory, Research, and Clinical Applications* (pp. 520–554). New York: Guilford.

Lyons-Ruth, K., Dutra, L., Schuder, M. and Boachi, I. (2006). From infant attachment disorganization to adult dissociation: relational adaptations or traumatic experience? *Psychiatric Clinics of North America*, 29, 63–86.

MacDonald, H. Z., Beeghly, M., Grant-Knight, W., Augustyn, M., Woods, R. W., Cabral, H., and Frank, D. A. (2008). Longitudinal association between infant disorganized attachment and childhood posttraumatic stress symptoms. *Development and Psychopathology*, 20 (2), 493–508. doi:10.1017/S0954579408000243

Macfie, J., Brumariu, L. E., and Lyons-Ruth, K. (2015). Parent–child role-confusion: A critical review of an emerging concept. *Developmental Review*, 36, 34–57. doi:10.1016/j.dr.2015.01.002

Madden, A. R., and Shaffer, A. (2016). Childhood parentification and adult relationship functioning. *Journal of Adult Development*, 23 (2), 90–102.

Mahler, M., Pine, S. and Bergmann, A. (1975). *The Psychological Birth of the Human Infant*. New York: Basic Books.

Main, M. and Goldwyn, S. (1995). Interview-based adult attachment classification: related to infant-mother and infant-father attachment. *Developmental Psychology*, 19, 237–223.

Main, M., and Hesse, E. (1990). Parents' unresolved traumatic experiences are related to infant disorganized attachment status: Is frightened and/or frightening parental behavior the linking mechanism? In M. T. Greenberg, D. Cicchetti, and E. M. Cummings (eds), *Attachment in the Preschool Years* (pp. 161–182). Chicago, IL: University of Chicago Press.

Main, M., and Solomon, J. (1986). Discovery of a new, insecure-disorganized/disoriented attachment pattern. In T. B. Brazelton and M. Yogman (eds), *Affective Development in Infancy* (pp. 95–124). Norwood: Ablex.

Main, M., Kaplan, N., and Cassidy, J. (1985). *Security in Infancy, Childhood, and Adulthood: A Move to the Level of Representation. Monographs of the Society for Research in Child Development*, 50 (1–2), 66–104.

Malach-Pines, A., and Yafe-Yenai, O. (1999). Unconscious influences on a choice of career: implications for organizational consultation. *Journal of Health and Human Services Administration*, 21 (4), 502–511.

Mardani, A., Jafari, E., Safari, Y., Khamnian, Z., and Alipour, F. (2023). Challenges in addiction-affected families: A systematic review of qualitative studies. *BMC Public Health*, 23, 989.

Maroda, K. J. (2022). *The Analyst's Vulnerability: Impact on Theory and Practice*. London/New York: Routledge.

Masiran, N. A., Ibrahim, N., Nik Jaafar, N. R., and Siau, C. S. (2023). The positive and negative aspects of parentification: An integrated review. *Frontiers in Psychology*, 14, 1159739.

Masson, J. M. (ed. and trans.). (1985). *The Complete Letters of Sigmund Freud to Wilhelm Fliess, 1887–1904*. Cambridge, MA: Harvard University Press.

Matthys F. (2000). *Leven met een verslaafde.* Antwerpen-Appeldoorn: Garant.

McDougall, J. (1989). *Les théâtres du corps.* Paris: Gallimard.

McWilliams, N. (2004). *Psychoanalytic Psychotherapy: A Practitioner's Guide.* New York: Guilford.

Mikulincer, M., and Shaver, P. R. (2016). *Attachment in Adulthood: Structure, Dynamics, and Change* (2nd edn). New York: Guilford.

Miller, A. (1979). *The Drama of the Gifted Child: The Search for the True Self* (3rd edn). New York: Basic Books, 2008.

Mintz, D. L. (2015). Teaching the prescriber's role: The psychology of psychopharmacology. *Academic Psychiatry*, 29 (2), 187–194. doi:10.1176/appi.ap.29.2.187

Minuchin, S. (1971). *Families and Family Therapy.* London/New York: Routledge, 1977.

Minuchin, S. (1981). *Family Therapy Techniques.* Cambridge, MA: Harvard University Press.

Minuchin, S. B. Montalvo, B. G. Guerney, B. Rosman, and F. Schumer (1976). *Families of the Slums: An Exploration of Their Structure and Treatment.* New York: Basic Books.

Mitchell, S. A. (1988). *Relational Concepts in Psychoanalysis: An Integration.* Cambridge, MA: Harvard University Press.

Mitchell, S. A., and Aron, L. (Eds.). (1999). *Relational Psychoanalysis: The Emergence of a Tradition.* New York: The Analytic Press.

Monjauze, M. (1999). *La part alcoolique du soi: la prise en charge clinique des patients alcooliques.* Paris: Dunod.

Monjauze, M. (2000). *Alcoolisme et processus psychiques.* Paris: Dunod.

Monjauze, M. (2004). L'alcoolisme: entre clivage et effondrement. *Revue Française de Psychanalyse*, 68 (5), 1617–1632.

Murphy, R. A., and Halgin, R. P. (1995). Influences on the career choice of psychotherapists. *Professional Psychology: Research and Practice*, 26, 422–425.

Napora, E. (2016). Parentification and grandparents' support from the perspective of grandchildren from families of various structures. *Acta Educationis Generalis*, 6 (1), 9–26.

Nehrig, N., Ho, S. S. M., and Wong, P. S. (2019). Understanding the self-object needs inventory: Its relationship to narcissism, attachment, and childhood maltreatment. *Psychoanalytic Psychology*, 36 (1), 53–63. doi:10.1037/pap0000182

Nicolai, N. (2009). Gedesorganiseerde gehechtheid. Van babyonderzoek tot behandeling. *Tijdschrift voor psychoanalyse*, 15, 16–28.

Nicolai, N. (2010) Parentificatie vanuit gehechtheidsperspectief. In M. Kinet (ed.) *Parentificatie. Als het kind te snel ouder wordt* (pp. 87–106). Antwerpen/Apeldoorn: Garant.

Nietzsche, F. (1908). *Ecce Homo – hoe iemand wordt wat hij is* (P. Hawinkels and P. Beers, vert.). Amsterdam/Antwerpen: de Arbeiderspers, 2005.

Norcross, J. C., and Farber, B. A. (2005). Choosing psychotherapy as a career: Beyond 'I want to help people.' *Journal of Clinical Psychology*, 61 (8), 939–943. doi:10.1002/jclp.20175

Norcross, J. C., and VandenBos, G. R. (2018). *Leaving it at the Office: A Guide to Psychotherapist Self-Care.* New York: Guilford.

Nuttall, A. K., Zhang, Q., Valentino, K., and Borkowski, J. G. (2019). Intergenerational risk of parentification and infantilization to externalizing moderated by child temperament. *Journal of Marriage and Family*, 81 (3), 648–661. doi:10.1111/jomf.12562

Ogden, T. H. (1986). *The Matrix of the Mind: Object Relations and the Psychoanalytic Dialogue*. New York: Jason Aronson.

Onderwaater, A. (2009). *De onverbrekelijke band. Inleiding & ontwikkelingen in de contextuele therapie van Nagy*. Amsterdam: Pearson.

Oppenoorth, W. (1990). Parentificatie en projectieve identificatie. *Tijdschrift voor Psychotherapie*, 16, 25–35.

Oppenoorth, W. (1994). Parentificatie als ouderlijke projectieve identificatie. *Gezinstherapie*, 6 (1), 13–29.

Ord, T. (2020). *The Precipice: Existential Risk and the Future of Humanity*. New York: Bloomsbury.

Orlinsky, D. E., and Rønnestad, M. H. (2005). *How Psychotherapists Develop: A Study of Therapeutic Work and Professional Growth*. Washington, DC: American Psychological Association.

Panksepp, J. (1998). *Affective Neuroscience: The Foundations of Human and Animal Emotions*. Oxford: Oxford University Press.

Park, S., and Schepp, K. G. (2015). A systematic review of research on children of alcoholics: Their inherent resilience and vulnerability. *Journal of Child and Family Studies*, 24 (5), 1222–1231. doi:10.1007/s10826-014-9930-7

Pasternak, A., and Schier, K. (2012). The role reversal in the families of Adult Children of Alcoholics. *Archives of Psychiatry and Psychotherapy*, 14 (3), 51–57.

Peirce, C. S. (1994), *Peirce on Signs: Writings on Semiotics* (J. Hoopes, ed.) Chapel Hill, NC: University of North Carolina Press.

Phillips, A. (1993). *On Kissing, Tickling, and Being Bored: Psychoanalytic Essays on the Unexamined Life*. Cambridge, MA: Harvard University Press.

Phillips, A. (2007). *Winnicott*. London: Penguin Books.

Priel, B., and Besser, A. (2001). Vulnerability to depression: The contribution of attachment styles and the regulation of self-worth. *Personality and Individual Differences*, 31 (5), 789–801.

Puchol-Martínez, F., Puchol-Ferrándiz, A., and Castellano-Tejedor, C. (2023). Preventive interventions for children and adolescents of parents with mental illness: A systematic review. *Clinical Psychology and Psychotherapy*, 30 (5), 979–997. doi:10.1002/cpp.2850

Råbu, M., Moltu, C., Binder, P. E., and McLeod, J. (2016). How does practicing psychotherapy affect the personal life of the therapist? A qualitative inquiry of senior therapists' experiences. *Psychotherapy Research*, 26 (6), 737–749. doi:10.1080/10503307.2015.1065354

Racker, H. (1968). *Transference and Countertransference*. London: Karnac, 1982.

Rado, S. (1926). The psychic effects of intoxicants: an attempt to evolve a psychoanalytical theory of morbid cravings. *Int. J. Psychoanal.*, XII, 396–413.

Rapa, E., Dodsworth, J., Ntuli, A., Anderson, J., Harper, G., and Stein, A. (2025). 'I don't know what to tell them': Experiences of patients talking about mental illness with children and how clinical teams can help. *Frontiers in Psychology*, 16, 1504130. doi:10.3389/fpsyg.2024.1504130

Reder, P., McClure, M., and Jolley, A. (2005). *Family Matters: Interfaces between Child and Adult Mental Health*. London/New York: Routledge.

Rek, I., Ehrenthal, J. C., Strauss, B. M., Schauenburg, H., Nikendei, C. and Dinger, U. (2018). Attachment styles and interpersonal motives of psychotherapy trainees. *Psychotherapy*, 55 (3), 209–215.

Rober, P. (1999). The therapist's inner conversation in family therapy practice: Some ideas about the self of the therapist, therapeutic impasse, and the process of reflection. *Family Process*, 38 (2), 209.

Rober, P. (2024). *Becoming an Effective Family Therapist: Research, Practice, and Case Stories.* London/New York: Routledge.

Rockland, L. H. (1989). *Supportive Therapy. A Psychodynamic Approach.* New York: Basic Books.

Rosenfeld, H. (1960). The psychopathology of drug addiction and alcoholism: a critical review of the psychoanalytic literature. *Psychotic States* (pp. 217–252). London: Hogarth Press, 1964.

Rosenfeld, H. (1964). On the psychopathology of narcissism: A clinical approach. *International Journal of Psychoanalysis*, 45, 332–337.

Rosenfeld, H. (1971). A clinical approach to the psychoanalytic theory of the life and death instinct: an investigation into the aggressive aspects of narcissism. *International Journal of Psycho-Analysis*, 52, 169–178.

Saha, A. (2016). Parentification: Boon or bane? *Journal of Psychological Research*, 11 (2), 289–301.

Sang, J., Cederbaum, J. A., and Hurlburt, M. S. (2014). Parentification, substance use, and sex among adolescent daughters from ethnic minority families. *Family Process*, 53 (2), 252–266. doi:10.1111/famp.12038

Santayana, G. (1905). *The Life of Reason: The Phases of Human Progress* (Vol. 1). New York: Scribners.

Satir, V. (1967). *Conjoint Family Therapy: A Guide to Theory and Technique.* Palo Alto, CA: Science and Behavior Books.

Satir, V. (1972). *Peoplemaking*. Palo Alto, CA: Science and Behavior Books, 1983.

Schier, K. (2012). The role reversal in the families of adult children of alcoholics. *Archives of Psychiatry and Psychotherapy*, 14 (3), pp. 51–57.

Schore, A. N. (1994). *Affect Regulation and the Origin of the Self.* New York: Erlbaum.

Schore, A. N. (2001). Effects of a secure attachment relationship on right brain development, affect regulation, and infant mental health. *Infant Mental Health Journal*, 22 (1–2), 7–66. doi:10.1002/1097-0355(200101/04)22:1

Schore, A. N. (2019). *Right Brain Psychotherapy.* New York: Norton.

Schore, A. N. (2021). *The Development of the Unconscious Mind.* New York: Norton.

Schorr, S., and Goldner, L. (2023). 'Like stepping on glass': A theoretical model to understand the emotional experience of childhood parentification. *Family Relations*, 72(5), 3029–3048.

Schuengel, C. (1997). Disorganized attachment in infancy: A review of the phenomenon and its implications for clinical practice. *Infant Mental Health Journal*, 18 (1), 3–19. doi:10.1002/(SICI)1097-0355(199721)18:1

Searles, H. F. (1965). The patient as psychiatrist to his analyst. In H. F. Searles, *Collected Papers on Schizophrenia and Related Subjects* (pp. 300–321). New York: International Universities Press.

Selvini Palazzoli, M., Boscolo, L., Cecchin, G., and Prata, G. (1980). Hypothesizing—circularity—neutrality: Three guidelines for the conductor of the session. *Family Process*, 19 (1), 3–12.

Shaver, P. R., Belsky, J. A. Y., and Brennan, K. A. (2000). The adult attachment interview and self-reports of romantic attachment: Associations across domains and methods. *Personal Relationships*, 7 (1), 25–43.

Shin, Y. J., and Hecht, M. L. (2013). Does parentification place Mexican-heritage youth at risk for substance use? Identifying the intervening nature of parent-child communication about alcohol. *Journal of Adolescence*, 36 (1), 149–159. doi:10.1016/j.adolescence.2012.10.010

Sklar, J. (2012). Regression and new beginnings: Michael, Alice and Enid Balint and the circulation of ideas. *International Journal of Psycho-Analysis*, 93 (4), 1017–1034. doi:10.1111/j.1745-8315.2012.00559.x

Skynner, R. and Cleese, J. (1986). *Families and How to Survive them*. London: Oxford University Press.

Slade, A. (2005). Parental reflective functioning: An introduction. *Attachment and Human Development*, 7 (3), 269–281. doi:10.1080/14616730500245906

Smith, J. A., Flowers, P., and Larkin, M. (2009). *Interpretative Phenomenological Analysis: Theory, Method and Research*. London: Sage.

Smith, P. L., and Moss, S. B. (2009). Psychologist impairment: What is it, how can it be prevented, and what can be done to address it? *Clinical Psychology: Science and Practice*, 16, 1–15. https://psycnet.apa.org/doi/10.1111/j.1468-2850.2009.01137.x

Sneller, R. (2020). Kierkegaard on Socrates' daimonion. *International Journal of Philosophy and Theology*, 81 (1), 87–100. doi:10.1080/21692327.2019.1649602

Solms, M. (2021). *The Hidden Spring: A Journey to the Source of Consciousness*. New York: Norton.

Solomon, J., and George, C. (1999). The measurement of attachment security in infancy and childhood. In J. Cassidy and P. R. Shaver (eds), *Handbook of Attachment: Theory, Research, and Clinical Applications* (pp. 287–316). New York: Guilford.

Staal, C. (2024). De psychotherapeut als wounded healer. *De Psycholoog*. April, pp. 11–18. https://www.tijdschriftdepsycholoog.nl/wetenschap/de-psychotherapeut-als-wounded-healer/

Steele, M., Kaniuk, J., Hodges, J, Asquith, K., Hillmann, and Steele, H. (2008). Measuring mentalization across contexts. In E. Jurist, A. Slade, and S. Bergner (eds), *Mind to Mind: Infant Research, Neuroscience and Psychoanalysis* (pp. 115–139). New York: Other Press.

Stein, G. L., Gonzalez, L. M., Cupito, A. M., Kiang, L., and Supple, A. J. (2015). The protective role of familism in the lives of Latino adolescents. *Journal of Family Issues*, 36(10), 1255–1273. doi:10.1177/0192513X13502480

Stern, D. N. (1985). *The Interpersonal World of the Infant*. New York: Basic Books.

Stuyt, A. (2007). Psychoanalyse en alcoholisme: Michèle Monjauze en haar klinische inzichten. *Tijdschrift voor Psychoanalyse*, 16 (1), 119–134.

Sussman, M. B. (1992). *A Curious Calling. Unconscious Motivations for Practising Psychotherapy*. Northvale, NJ; London: Jason Aronson.

Symington, N. (1986). *The Analytic Experience: Lectures from the Tavistock*. London: Free Association Books.

Taillieu, T. L., Brownridge, D. A., Sareen, J., and Afifi, T. O. (2016). Childhood emotional maltreatment and mental disorders: Results from a nationally representative adult sample from the United States. *Child Abuse & Neglect*, 59, 1–12. doi:10.1016/j.chiabu.2016.07.005

Tedgård, E., Råstam, M., and Wirtberg, I. (2019). An upbringing with substance-abusing parents: Experiences of parentification and dysfunctional communication. *NAD Nordic Studies on Alcohol and Drugs*, 36 (3), 223–247. doi:10.1177/1455072518814308

Thastum, M., Johansen, M. B., Gubba, L., Olesen, L. B., and Romer, G. (2008). Coping, social relations, and communication: A qualitative exploratory study of children of parents with cancer. *Clinical Child Psychology and Psychiatry*, 13 (1), 123–138. doi:10.1177/1359104507086345

Thys, M. (2010). Tussen nijd en spijt. Parentificatie en reparatie. In M. Kinet (ed.) *Parentificatie. Als het kind te snel ouder wordt* (pp. 59–86). Antwerpen/Apeldoorn: Garant.

Thys, M. (2015) Projectieve identificatie tussen doodsdrift en intersubjectiviteit. *Tijdschrift voor Psychoanalyse*, 2, 83–97.

Titzmann, P. F. (2012). Growing up too soon? Parentification among immigrant and native adolescents in Germany. *Journal of Youth and Adolescence*, 41, 880–893. doi:10.1007/s10964-011-9711-1

Tompkins, T. L. (2007). Parentification and maternal HIV infection: Beneficial role or pathological burden? *Journal of Child and Family Studies*, 16 (1), 108–118. doi:10.1007/s10826–10006–9072–9077

Tronick, E. (2007). *The Neurobehavioral and Social-Emotional Development of Infants and Children*. New York: Norton.

Tronick, E., Als, H., Adamson, L., Wise, S., and Brazelton, T. B. (1978). The infant's response to entrapment between contradictory messages in face-to-face interaction. *Journal of the American Academy of Child Psychiatry*, 17 (1), 1–13.

Valleau, M. P., Bergner, R. M., and Horton, C. B. (1995). Parentification and caretaker syndrome: An empirical investigation. *Family Therapy*, 22 (3), 157–164.

Van Buren, B. R., and Meehan, K. B. (2015). Child maltreatment and vulnerable narcissism: The roles of shame and disavowed need. *Journal of the American Psychoanalytic Association*, 63 (3), 555–561. doi:10.1177/0003065115593058

Van den Eerenbeemt, E.-M. (2016). *Door het oog van de familie*. Amsterdam: Balans.

Van der Kolk, B. A. (2014). *The Body Keeps the Score: Brain, Mind, and Body in the Healing of Trauma*. New York: Viking.

Van der Pas, A., and De Ruiter, E. (1992). *Parentificatie: Een contextueel perspectief*. Utrecht: SWP.

Van Gael, M. (1998). Als de chirurg in eigen vingers snijdt. Over de grenzen van de draagkracht van de psychotherapeut. *Tijdschrift voor Psychotherapie*, 24, 28–35.

Van Gael, M. (2000). Is de therapeut 'vrij van herinnering en verlangen?' *Tijdschrift Klinische Psychologie*, 30 (1), 4–12.

Van Gael, M. (2020). Als de chirurg in eigen vingers snijdt – anno 2020. *Tijdschrift voor Psychotherapie*, 46 (3), 151–164.

Van Haute, P. (2000). *Tegen de aanpassing*. Nijmegen: SUN.

Van IJzendoorn, M. H. (1994). *Gehechtheid tussen ouders en kinderen*. Houten: Bohn Stafleu Van Loghum.

Van IJzendoorn, M. H. and Bakemans-Kranenburg, M. H. (2008). The distribution of adult attachment representations in clinical groups. Metanalytic search for patterns in attachment. In H. Steele and M. Steele (eds), *Clinical Applications of the Adult Attachment Interview* (pp. 69–96). New York: Guilford.

Van IJzendoorn, M. H., and Bakermans-Kranenburg, M. J. (2019). Bridging the transmission gap: What attachment measures can teach us. *Attachment and Human Development*, 21 (4), 402–409.

Van Loon, L. M. A., Van de Ven, M. O. M., Van Doesum, K. T. M., Hosman, C. M. H., and Witteman, C. L. M. (2017). Parentification, stress, and problem behavior of adolescents who have a parent with mental health problems. *Family Process*, 56 (1), 141–153. doi:10.1111/famp.12165

Van Mierlo, F., Michielsen, M., De Buysser, M. and Rooijakkers-Segers, G. (1998). Passend geven en nemen: hulpverlening aan volwassenen die als kind geparentificeerd werden. In M. Michielsen, W. van Mulligen and L. Hermkens (eds), *Leren over leven in loyaliteit. Over contextuele hulpverlening* (83–107). Leuven/Amersfoort: Acco.

Van Schoors, M., Van Lierde, E., Steeman, K., Verhofstadt, L. L., and Lemmens, G. M. (2023). Protective factors enhancing resilience in children of parents with a mental illness: A systematic review. *Frontiers in Psychology*, 14, 1243784. doi:10.3389/fpsyg.2023.1243784

Vandermeeren, R. (2004). Psychoanalytische reflecties over zelf en object in alcoholisme. *Tijdschrift voor psychoanalyse* 10, 135–147.

Vanheule, S., and Verhaeghe, P. (2004). Narcisme, alcoholisme en tegenoverdracht. *Tijdschrift voor Psychoanalyse*, 10 (2), 133–150.

Velleman, R., and Templeton, L. J. (2016). Impact of parents' substance misuse on children: an update. *BJPsych Advances*, 22 (2), 108–117. doi:10.1192/apt.bp.114.014449

Verhaeghe, P. (2002). *Over normaliteit en andere afwijkingen*. Leuven/Leusden: Acco.

Verhaeghe, P. (2009) *Het einde van de psychotherapie*. Amsterdam: Bezige Bij.

Verheul R., and van den Brink W. (1999). Persoonlijkheidsstoornissen. In: de Jong A., van den Brink W., Ormel J. and Wiersma D. (eds), *Handboek psychiatrische epidemiologie*. Maarsden: Elsevier/de Tijdstroom.

Von Bertalanffy, L. (1968). *General System Theory*. New York: Braziller.

Wallin, D. (2007). *Attachment in Psychotherapy*. New York: Guilford.

Wang, M., Liu, S., and Belsky, J. (2017). Triangulation processes experienced by children in contemporary China. *International Journal of Behavioral Development*, 41 (6), 688–695. doi:10.1177/0165025416662345

Watzlawick, P., Beavin, J. H., and Jackson, D. D. (1967). *Pragmatics of Human Communication: A Study of Interactional Patterns, Pathologies, and Paradoxes*. New York: Norton.

Wegscheider-Cruse, S. (1989). *Another Chance: Hope and Health for the Alcoholic Family*. Palo Alto, CA: Science and Behavior Books.

West, M. L., and Keller, A. E. (1991). Parentification of the child: A case study of Bowlby's compulsive care-giving attachment pattern. *American Journal of Psychotherapy*, 45 (3), 425–431.

Westman, J., Jayaram-Lindström, N., Kane, K., Franck, J., and Gissler, M. (2022). Mortality in adult children of parents with alcohol use disorder: A nationwide register study. *European Journal of Epidemiology*, 37 (8), 815–826. doi:10.1007/s10654-022-00883-4

Whitaker, C. A., and Bumberry, W. M. (1988). *Dancing with the Family: A Symbolic-Experiential Approach*. New York: Brunner/Mazel.

Widom, C. S. (1993). Child abuse and alcohol use and abuse. In: Martin, S. E. (ed.), *Alcohol and Interpersonal Violence: Fostering Multidisciplinary Perspectives* (pp. 291–314). Rockville, MD: National Institute on Alcohol Abuse and Alcoholism.

Wikipedia (n.d.a). 'Salvador Minuchin.' *Wikipedia*. Available at: https://en.wikipedia.org/wiki/Salvador_Minuchin

Wikipedia (n.d.b). 'Ivan Boszormenyi-Nagy.' *Wikipedia*. Available at: https://en.wikipedia.org/wiki/Ivan_Boszormenyi-Nagy

Williams, K., and Francis, S. E. (2010). Parentification and psychological adjustment: Locus of control as a moderating variable. *Contemporary Family Therapy*, 32(3), 231–237. doi:10.1007/s10591-010-9123-5

Winer, J. (1994). The parentified therapist. *Contemporary Psychoanalysis*, 30 (2), 297–314.

Winnicott, D. W. (1939). Aggression and its roots. In C. Winnicott, R. Shepherd, and M. Davis (eds), *Deprivation and Delinquency* (pp. 86–94). London: Tavistock, 1984.

Winnicott, D. W. (1945). Primitive emotional development. *Through Paediatrics to Psycho-analysis* (pp. 145–156). London: Karnac, 1992.

Winnicott, D. W. (1947). Hate in the countertransference. *Through Paediatrics to Psycho-analysis* (pp. 194–203). London: Hogarth, 1958.

Winnicott, D. W. (1950). Some thoughts on the meaning of the word 'democracy.' In C. Winnicott, R. Shepherd, and M. Davis (eds), *Home is Where We Start From: Essays by a Psychoanalyst* (pp. 50–54). London: Penguin, 1986.

Winnicott, D. W. (1951). Transitional objects and transitional phenomena. In: *Through Paediatrics to Psycho-analysis* (pp. 229–242). London: Hogarth, 1958.

Winnicott, D. W. (1954). Metapsychological and clinical aspects of regression within the psycho-analytical set-up. *Through Paediatrics to Psycho-analysis* (pp. 278–294). London: Hogarth, 1958.

Winnicott, D. W. (1955–1956). Clinical varieties of transference. *Through Paediatrics to Psycho-analysis* (pp. 295–299). London: Hogarth, 1958.

Winnicott, D. W. (1956). Primary maternal preoccupation. *International Journal of Psycho-Analysis*, 37, 586–595. *Through Paediatrics to Psycho-analysis* (pp. 300–305). London: Hogarth, 1958.

Winnicott, D. W. (1958). The capacity to be alone. *International Journal of Psycho-Analysis*, 39, 416–420. *The Maturational Processes and the Facilitating Environment* (pp. 29–36). London: Hogarth, 1965.

Winnicott, D. W. (1960). The theory of the parent-infant relationship. *International Journal of Psycho-Analysis*, 41, 585–595. *The Maturational Processes and the Facilitating Environment* (pp. 37–55). London: Hogarth, 1965.

Winnicott, D. W. (1960). Ego distortion in terms of true and false self. *The Maturational Processes and the Facilitating Environment* (pp. 140–152). London: Hogarth, 1965.

Winnicott, D. W. (1962). Ego integration in child development. In *The Maturational Processes and the Facilitating Environment* (pp. 56–63). London: Hogarth, 1965.

Winnicott, D. W. (1963). From dependence towards independence in the development of the individual. *The Maturational Processes and the Facilitating Environment* (pp. 83–92). London: Hogarth, 1965.

Winnicott, D. W. (1963). The development of the capacity for concern. *Bulletin of the Menninger Clinic*, 27 (4), 167.

Winnicott, D. W. (1965). *The Maturational Processes and the Facilitating Environment: Studies in the Theory of Emotional Development*. London: Hogarth.

Winnicott, D. W. (1968). Communication between infant and mother, and mother and infant, compared and contrasted. *Babies and Their Mothers* (pp. 89–103). Reading, MA: Addison-Wesley, 1987.

Winnicott, D. W. (1968). The use of an object and relating through identifications. *International Journal of Psycho-Analysis*, 49, 585–595.

Winnicott, D. W. (1969). Symposium on envy and jealousy. *Psychoanalytic Explorations* (pp. 224–231). London: Karnac, 1989.

Winnicott, D. W. (1969). The mother–infant experience of mutuality. *Psychoanalytic Explorations* (pp. 215–223). London: Karnac, 1989.

Winnicott, D. W. (1971). *Playing and Reality*. London: Tavistock.

Winnicott, D. W. (1974). Fear of breakdown. *International Review of Psycho-analysis*, 1 (1–2), 103–107.

Winnicott, D. W. (1986). *Holding and Interpretation: Fragment of an Analysis*. London: Karnac, 1989.

Woititz, J. G. (1983). *Adult Children of Alcoholics*. Deerfield Beach, FL: Health Communications.

World Health Organisation. (2018). *Global Status Report on Alcohol and Health 2018*. Geneva: WHO.

Wrzesniewski, A., McCauley, C., Rozin, P., and Schwartz, B. (1997). Jobs, careers, and callings: People's relations to their work. *Journal of Research in Personality*, 31(1), 21–33.

Yew, S. G. K., Low, W. Y., and Tong, S. F. (2017). The influence of parentification on the well-being of adolescents in Malaysia. *Journal of Family Issues*, 38(13), 1848–1869. doi:10.1177/0192513X15598542

Young-Bruehl, E. (2002). A visit to the Budapest School. *The Psychoanalytic Study of the Child*, 57, 411–432.

Zerubavel, N., and Wright, M. O. (2012). The dilemma of the wounded healer. *Psychotherapy*, 49 (4), 482–491.

Žižek, S. (1992). *Enjoy Your Symptom! Jacques Lacan in Hollywood and Out*. London/New York: Routledge.

Index

For Product Safety Concerns and Information please contact our EU representative GPSR@taylorandfrancis.com Taylor & Francis Verlag GmbH, Kaufingerstraße 24, 80331 München, Germany